THE FUTURE OF
HEALTH-CARE
DELIVERY

Also by Stephen C. Schimpff, MD

The Future of Medicine: Megatrends in Health Care
That Will Improve Your Quality of Life (2007)

Alignment: The Key to the Success of the University of Maryland
Medical System (2009), with Morton I. Rapoport, MD

THE FUTURE OF
HEALTH-CARE
DELIVERY

*Why It
Must Change
and How It
Will Affect You*

Stephen C. Schimpff, MD

Potomac Books
Washington, D.C.

Information contained in this book, or in any other publication, article, or website cited herein, should not be considered a substitute for consultation with a board-certified physician to address individual medical needs. The author of *The Future of Health-Care Delivery*, Stephen C. Schimpff, MD, and the publisher, Potomac Books, disclaim any liability, loss, or damage that might result from the implementation of the contents of this book.

Library of Congress Cataloging-in-Publication Data
Schimpff, Stephen C., 1941–
  The future of health-care delivery : why it must change and how it will affect you / Stephen C. Schimpff.—1st ed.
     p. cm.
  Includes bibliographical references and index.
  ISBN 978-1-61234-156-9 (hardcover)
  ISBN 978-1-61234-157-6 (electronic edition)
  1. Medical care—United States—Forecasting. 2. Medical policy—United States—Forecasting. I. Title.
  RA395.A3S3664 2012
  362.101'12—dc23

                                    2011041710

Printed in the United States of America on acid-free paper that meets the American National Standards Institute Z39-48 Standard.

Potomac Books
22841 Quicksilver Drive
Dulles, Virginia 20166

First Edition

10 9 8 7 6 5 4 3 2 1

To Carol,
wife, best friend, and soul mate

CONTENTS

PREFACE

In the early 2000s I was invited to speak to a Chamber of Commerce group on what they titled "The Future of Medicine." Left to decide what the title meant, I chose to talk about the exciting scientific and technical advances in medicine that are revolutionizing care and will do so in the next five to fifteen years. I included areas such as genomics, stem cells, vaccines, transplantation, medical devices, imaging, and the operating room. To my pleasure, the audience was most interested and kept me for an extended question-and-answer session. Soon I began receiving requests to give similar talks to many groups and, given the interest, decided to put these thoughts into writing after I retired as CEO of the University of Maryland Medical Center. So was born *The Future of Medicine: Megatrends in Health Care That Will Improve Your Quality of Life*. But as I gave talks, invariably the questioners afterward asked about the rapidly rising costs of health care; about access to insurance; about frustrations with their doctor, hospital, or insurance company; and about why so many Americans do not have good health, good health-care coverage, or both. In short, they wanted to know what was wrong with the *delivery* of medical care and what could be done to improve it. And why do we focus on medical care rather than the totality of all the elements that would lead to health preservation and, when necessary, its restoration? These insistent and persistent questions led me to begin work on this book.

To develop the background information, I interviewed more than 150 leaders from across the country: hospital CEOs, chief operating officers, chief information officers, and chief financial officers, along with vice presidents of nursing and medical affairs, pharmacy directors, emergency room directors, and laboratory directors; physicians in academic and private practices; senior leaders at national organizations such as the American Hospital Association and the American Association of Medical Colleges; leaders in the insurance industry; health-care consultants, politicians, and their staff members; and others. They each had their own perspectives and some were certainly parochial, suggesting that an industry or group other than their own was at fault for the health-care industry's current problems. But their observations and recommendations were remarkably consistent. I also reviewed current literature on the topics and updated it by conducting further interviews and attending professional and scientific meetings.

After bringing all of this information together, I distilled it to the basic principles, as I see them, and organized them into a coherent whole that became this book.

We can expect innovations in biomedical, engineering, and computer science to bring potentially revolutionary changes. But not well appreciated are the other changes to medical care delivery that are coming as a result of an aging population, our adverse lifestyles and our behaviors, a coming shortage of providers, our attitudes about the end of life, and a nascent rise in consumerism.

There are also many misconceptions that exist about what medical care delivery is and what it could and should be. Few people understand that true health care requires an intensive focus not only on diagnosing and treating disease and injury when it occurs, but also on promoting health and preventing disease. A common misconception is that the health-care reform legislation will offer us better care opportunities, when in fact health-care reform is not about *health care*; it is mostly about *paying* for it: about providing medical care to the uninsured, about eliminating some of the health insurance restrictions consumers face, and only somewhat about the rising costs of medical care. It is more about expanding coverage, and when faced with the choice between expanding coverage and lowering cost, the federal government has pursued expanding coverage as the main goal.

Another misconception is that dealing with the financing system to create universal coverage for all Americans will reduce costs. Unfortunately that is not the case; indeed it will substantially add expenditures. And the demand for more doctors will increase to provide care for the newly covered. It is also frequently stated that health-care costs will be reduced if we have an electronic medical record (EMR). No doubt an EMR will be exceedingly valuable for patient care quality and safety, but it will be difficult to implement and is not likely to reduce costs much. We are also led to believe that health-care reform will reduce the costs of care or of insurance, yet it is unlikely that these goals will be reached.

These misconceptions that have developed over recent years are intriguing because the real information is actually available, yet few seem to realize or understand it. In this book I will explain the coming disruptions to care delivery and clarify the facts regarding common misconceptions. I will then offer specific recommendations that America needs to take to move from a health-care system that treats disease and injury to one that focuses on health promotion and disease prevention and provides coordinated care to those with complex, chronic illnesses.

To accomplish this goal requires fundamental changes in how we pay for medical care, how we fund preventive medicine and public health, how we manage medical information, how we incentivize and pay health-care providers, how we motivate ourselves to take better care of our health, and how we ensure that everyone in this great country has both access to care and the means to pay for it. It will mean reorganizing medical care so that the consumer is the decision maker, as in any other industry or professional-customer relationship. In short, we need a major overhaul of the entire system that *realigns incentives and balances fundamental rights with corresponding responsibilities*. This transformation, of course, will only come incrementally and only with extensive effort on the part of many individual leaders in government, industry, and medicine.

There are many constraints and barriers to success, not the least of which are the physicians, the hospitals, and the pharmaceutical and medical device manufacturers who will be concerned that their revenue might decline and their power evaporate. The insurers and the government payers will resist the need to create monetary incentives for better care, feeling uncertain that it will result in lower total costs. And, yes, even the patients—you and I—will resist change, including resisting any perceived reduction in benefits from our insurance or any requirements to accept further responsibility to manage our own health; yet we individuals must take responsibility for our own and our family's health.

Despite the challenges, this work can be done, should be done, and indeed must be done, or else we will continue to be a country deficient in the care that everyone could and should have while expending more on a per capita basis than do other countries with equal or better health quality measures. Will this effort require spending huge new sums of money? No, as long as we follow the proper course, although the transition may well require added expenditures. Indeed, plenty of money is in the system now; the system needs to be reorganized so that the funds can be spent efficiently and effectively in a manner that will actually improve the quality of care while reducing the associated costs. All parties will need to accept responsibilities along with their rights, a view that is not prevalent today. Making these adjustments will be a major task, for sure, but it is certainly not insurmountable.

This overhaul of our current health-care delivery system sounds like a major task—and it is. But it is doable, and doable now. If we are successful, we can model world-class care that will be the standard other countries will emulate.

These three key themes—the disruptive changes that are coming and needed, the clarification of misconceptions, and the balancing of rights with responsibilities—will lead us to a superior health-care system that functions for the benefit of all.

PART I

A VISION FOR HEALTH-CARE DELIVERY IN THE TWENTY-FIRST CENTURY

Let's begin with an overview of the American health-care system—what is good and, unfortunately, what is not so good. Then we will examine the current misconceptions and myths of health care and health-care reform and compare them to what really needs to be done to improve health care for all in America.

1

The Difference between Health Care and Medical Care

We Americans like to pride ourselves on having the best health-care system in the world, but unfortunately that is not the case. We have a medical (that is, sick) care system—a system that waits until we become ill before it kicks into action—instead of a health-care system focused on helping us stay healthy. We give lip service to prevention and, depending on your definition, spend only about 1–3 percent of our $2 trillion in medical expenditures on public health.

By many measures, we do not rate favorably when compared to other industrialized societies. Our behavior and lifestyle make us prone to illnesses that are chronic, complex, lifelong, and life shortening, all of which make them very expensive to treat. That $2 trillion is by far more than other nations spend on a per capita basis. We spend almost $8,000 per person per year, about 50 percent more than the next closest developed country, and this expenditure is seriously and adversely affecting businesses, government, and each of us.[1] Employers complain that medical insurance reduces profits, and the fact is, it reduces wages, since businesses set a limit on employees' total compensation. If benefits including medical insurance are high, then wages will be correspondingly lower. It is a zero-sum game. The government cannot afford what it has promised, either: witness the current debate recently begun in Congress regarding the costs of Medicare. And each of us complains bitterly that the cost of care is too high—and that we cannot do anything about it.

Meanwhile, we may be pleased with our doctor but not with the health-care delivery system as a whole. Quality is subpar, preventable errors are rampant, and some 47 million Americans are without insurance or access to medical care. The United States is the only industrialized country to have this problem. Of course, we need to recognize that having insurance is not the same as having access to a physician; it is only the means to pay if one can find a provider. Politicians and the media focus on the access issues predominantly, cost issues somewhat, and the issues of quality, safety, and prevention and public health only rarely.

In *The Future of Medicine*, I wrote about my maternal grandfather who was a general practitioner in New York State. He graduated from medical school in 1898. He set up his practice in Beacon, a small town on the Hudson River in New York. He built a room on the side of his home to serve as his office and used the large wraparound front porch as the waiting room. There were no appointments; patients came and sat on the porch until it was their turn. Office hours lasted until the last patient had been seen and cared for. Initially there was no hospital, and he treated all patients in the office or at their home, although later in his career he helped establish a hospital directly across the street.

In his day a physician had relatively few tools with which to treat someone; the important part was to make a diagnosis and inform the patient and the family what the situation was and what the course of that illness would probably be like. Yes, my grandfather could provide some care, including treating pain with morphine, removing an inflamed appendix, sewing up lacerations, and delivering babies much more safely than could have been done without the assistance of a trained clinician. But during the course of his practice, which ended with his death in 1936, medicine began to change toward a much more scientific basis. To a large degree it was propelled by the influence of Johns Hopkins University School of Medicine and Hospital in Baltimore, Maryland. Founded in the late 1800s, it instituted the concept that medicine was and should be a science and taught a science-based medical program during four years of medical school plus practical training, establishing what we know today as the standard residency training program following medical school. This approach brought about a dramatic change in the way physicians thought about medicine and patient care.

In the course of his practice my grandfather saw the beginnings of those changes. Insulin was discovered in the 1920s, the first antibiotics in the 1930s. After his death and the completion of World War II, the National Institutes of Health (NIH) began to develop, grow, and distribute large sums of money across the country to various medical schools and within its own organization to conduct basic biomedical research. The result is that today our ability to repair, restore to function, or replace an organ, tissue, or cell has moved ahead at a dramatic pace and will do so even more quickly in the coming years. Concurrently, the pharmaceutical industry became scientific as well, resulting in a continual outpouring of new drugs that can relieve suffering, reverse harm, and cure many diseases while extending our life span. With the advent of the science of genomics, it is increasingly possible to predict the onset of disease before it occurs and thereby create a preventive approach for the individual patient. Soon we will have immediate access at any time and any place to our medical records, which will be fully digitized, and safety and quality of medical care will dramatically improve. All of this advancement occurred because of the shift to science-based medicine that was introduced only a hundred years ago.

Another change has happened. This change is very important but it has not been appreciated. In the past, illnesses tended to be "acute," meaning that they occurred and were treated, and the patients either got better or died. If your child developed strep throat, the pediatrician prescribed an antibiotic, and it got better. If you developed appendicitis, then your doctor referred you to a surgeon who operated and threw away the inflamed appendix, and you were cured. But today, most illnesses are chronic and complex. If a man survives a heart attack, he may still have some damaged heart muscle and so develops heart failure. This condition will be with him for life and will need multiple treatments, many medications, and probably a number of hospitalizations with a stay in the intensive care unit (ICU). It might even get to the point of his needing a heart transplant. Other examples are diabetes, rheumatoid arthritis, many cancers, chronic lung disease, kidney failure, and so many other diseases seen frequently today. This major shift enormously impacts how we should (but mostly do not) organize the treatment of the patient and his or her disease, how we should (but mostly do not) organize the payment system for that care, how we should (but mostly do not) use technologies wisely for care, and how we should (but mostly do not) ensure quality and safety in patient care. This change is profound, but most of the approaches to health-care reform do not address the implications of this shift to chronic, complex, lifelong illness, perhaps because it has not been well recognized. Although they are aware of the change toward more and more chronic illnesses, physicians, too, tend to want to preserve their current practice methods, which were developed over the years to handle the simpler acute illnesses, even though the current chronic and complex illnesses require a different approach.

In that same time frame of scientific advancement and the rising frequency of chronic illnesses, we also began to lose in medicine the true connection between the physician and the patient. Most of us patients feel as if we do not get to spend enough time with our physicians. They seem busy and distracted and not able or willing to listen to our stories. From the physician's perspective, he or she feels that there is not enough time to spend with an individual patient, not enough time to learn about the family and the environment in which that patient lives and therefore in which the patient's disease has occurred, and not enough time to focus on preventive instructions or to even talk fully about the plan for caring for a specific illness or problem. Instead, too much time is spent following mandates and filling out forms, often repeatedly; and then they are being paid well less than what their time and effort were worth.

All of those assertions are true, but a new force in medicine will add a set of dramatic changes—the force of consumerism. No longer will I, as a patient, be willing to be "patient." I will expect my caregiver to be responsive, prompt, effective, efficient, and, notably, both polite and professional. I will expect an adequate period of time with my caregiver and that the caregiver will get to know me as a person and indeed as a person who is part of a family, a community, and a society. I will not tolerate any longer being treated as a "number," a "case," or a "problem." If I don't receive the care in the manner I described, then I will seek out care elsewhere.

I saw an example of this expectation in a friend who developed breast cancer. After being seen immediately by a top-notch surgeon who did her biopsy and then lumpectomy in a very timely manner with plenty of discussion and hand-holding, she then went to a highly regarded medical oncologist with the expectation that she would receive her drug therapy and radiation therapy at that individual's hospital. She knew that the oncologist was well trained and competent. The physician seemed pleasant enough, but she was not engaging and not really focused on my friend as a person. It seemed as though she went though a checklist of information in a "rote-like" manner. The patient felt as if she was regarded as one more breast cancer patient rather than as an individual person who also had a particular problem. While she felt that perhaps the physician might have been having a tough day or that she, the patient, was being seen at the end of a long line of other patients that day, it was no matter. This physician was to be her primary caregiver for an issue that was of the utmost importance to her. The result was that my friend went elsewhere for both her medical oncology and her radiation therapy care. The basic message, of course, is that patients now want and expect not only competency, but also personal, professional care and that they will both pay for it and demand it.

Compare that story to this one. A couple went to a small Caribbean island for a two-week vacation. On the last day of their vacation the husband had a heart attack. He was taken to the island's small, twenty-five-bed hospital. He and his wife, who works at a major hospital in a patient care-advocacy profession, were immediately concerned that the level of care would not be up to the standards that they would have expected in their large U.S. city. To their obvious pleasure, his caregiver was a highly skilled physician who also interacted with both of them. He did the appropriate diagnostic tests to demonstrate that indeed it was a heart attack and then began the appropriate medical therapy. Concurrently he arranged the patient's air transport to a major hospital in Florida. Meanwhile, others at this small hospital helped the patient's wife not only to cope with her concerns, but also to deal with some of the practical issues of checking out of the hotel, returning the rental car, arranging for the medical evacuation flight, and attending to all the other myriad details. In short, they looked after her as well as her husband. She cannot speak highly enough of the care that her husband received.

Both of these stories also illustrate the issue of complex, chronic disease. Such diseases do not go away, and while they can be cured, the possibility of a subsequent problem (heart failure) or recurrence (cancer) is real. Many chronic illnesses will be with the patient for life. They require many different practitioners with differing skills, which all need to be coordinated, to care for them. But in America today, the care for these complex, chronic illnesses, which consume more than 70 percent of all medical care expenditures, is definitely not addressed in a coordinated manner— except in a few centers and practices. This lack of coordination of chronic illness care means that the care is not up to its potential quality levels, given our knowledge base and our excellent practitioners, and that the costs are much too high. The expenditures rise because patients are shuttled to too many specialists, receive unneeded tests and X-rays, and may even undergo unneeded procedures. We need to find a way to change our delivery system so that it delivers coordinated, compassionate, and safe care to individuals with these complex, chronic diseases.

Are we coming full circle? I think so. In my grandfather's day interpersonal skills with the patient were paramount. Knowing the patient, the patient's family, and where the patient lived was integral to understanding the disease that occurred in the patient. Indeed, it was important in those days to think of the patient as having a disease as opposed to a disease that had occurred in a patient. But in the second half of the twentieth century, as the medical profession became more and more scientifically based, a doctor tended to look at test results first and then do a brief history and physical exam with his or her mind already made up about the problem. Too often the focus was on the disease, not the patient. But that personal focus is essential for good care of the patient and especially for the patient with a chronic illness.

At the same time, our mechanism for reimbursement of care changed as well. No longer did individuals pay for their care directly, but rather through an intermediary—the insurance company, or a "third-party payer" (TTP)—with the cost of the insurance paid to a large degree by their employer if they were working or by Medicare if they were retired. So a disconnect occurred between the doctor and patient in that the patient no longer contracted directly with the physician for his or her service, paying only about 19 percent out of pocket. About 85 percent of Americans have medical care insurance, but because of the methods used to pay for it, most Americans have little comprehension of its real cost—that is, the total cost of the insurance and of the reduced wages resultant from the increasing cost of the insurance. At the same time, all physicians, but especially primary care physicians (PCPs), found that their incomes were either staying flat or declining yet their costs were increasing, their paperwork was going up dramatically, and their frustrations were beginning to outweigh the joys of patient care. More physicians became specialists, in part because of the glamour of the specialty but in large part also because the remuneration was better. Many will say the choice was dictated at least in part by large debts they incurred in medical school and in training.

Now patients are once again expected to assume a higher level of responsibility. We are now responsible for an increasing proportion of our insurance payments; they are no longer fully paid by our employer or Medicare—neither of which can afford it. We are faced with high deductibles and co-pays, and we are increasingly becoming responsible for our own health—as we should be. Still, there is a large disconnect between the dollars we expend and the care we receive, a disconnect that keeps us from effectively managing the dollars spent on our medical care. At the same time, we consumers increasingly expect quality, safety, professionalism, and responsiveness and are willing to look elsewhere for care if our expectations are not met. Still, if we are not directly contracting with our provider—either the doctor or the hospital—it is hard to hold the provider accountable. The consumer is *not the customer* in this model.

Physicians must coordinate the care of individuals with complex, chronic illnesses. No longer will it be sufficient to refer patients from one doctor to another. Too much information is lost, not enough quality is rendered, and too many excess tests, imaging, and procedures are performed. Our system of autonomous, independent practitioners will have to change to groups of physicians and other providers, or teams, each with their own skill sets, who will work together to care for a patient with a given problem. Certain large groups have demonstrated that they can dispense higher quality care at less expense for patients with complex, chronic illnesses. Individual PCPs can as well, provided they take on the responsibility to actually coordinate care. But this additional duty requires a change in their financial incentives.

Many PCPs—family medicine practitioners, pediatricians, internists—have opted not to accept insurance, especially Medicare. They simply expect their patients to pay them out of pocket for their care. My own internist and many others who I know personally have opted for "retainer-based" or "concierge" practices. In brief, I am required to pay my internist $1,500 per year. In return, the doctor will limit his practice to five hundred patients rather than the previous thirteen hundred patients, and he will guarantee that I can be seen within twenty-four hours of a call and that I will receive as much time as needed to address my problem. He will do a comprehensive annual exam, appropriate blood tests, and an electrocardiogram as indicated and administer routine immunizations. The doctor will meet me if I need to go to the emergency room (ER) and will do home visits or nursing home visits if the need arises. Depending on the physician's type of retainer practice, it means that the doctor will no longer bill the insurance company and so will no longer be hampered by the insurers' delays, turmoil, frustrations, or the low reimbursement payments that drive the doctor to see so many patients today simply to make ends meet.

Of course, this arrangement is a new and added expense for me at a time when, in semi-retirement, we are living mostly on our savings and limiting our expenditures. Given that the recent financial and stock market crises reduced those savings, it is a new cost burden that we did not want or expect. Indeed, it increases our total outlay for health care because we still need our insurance for specialists, procedures, imaging, drugs, and possible hospitalizations. Together, my wife and I already pay almost $8,000 per year for health-care insurance (despite the fact that Medicare Part A is "free"). Now we will be paying the doctor's retainer fee. I do not have any serious medical conditions today, but should one develop my hope and expectation is that my internist will have the time, the interest, and the inclination to coordinate fully and properly the care I will need from many specialists, centers, and institutions. That will be the real test of the system's value. It will be an interesting experiment; I hope we will not need to test it out soon. But this development should never have happened or have been necessary; it is a response to a broken reimbursement system.

So we have a delivery system that is largely focused on medical care, or diagnosing and treating disease once it occurs. We have incredible assets, including well-trained professionals, new knowledge about illnesses, remarkable new drugs and medical devices, and high-quality hospitals, clinics, and other support organizations. But we are not giving attention to prevention. In short, we have a medical care, not a health-care, system.

This point brings me to the major health-care political issue of the day, health-care reform. It has become the talk of Washington. Indeed, the average American now says that medical costs are so high that they compete with basic necessities and are getting to the point of being unaffordable. Americans want and need some form of action to make health-care costs more reasonable.

But what really is health-care reform all about? Is it about getting better medical care? More preventive care? Less bureaucracy when dealing with your insurance company? Less expensive medicines? Easier access to your physician or a specialist or a test or a procedure? Lower co-pays and deductibles? Is it about improving your health and well-being?

Unfortunately, not really. Reform in Washington is about how America should finance medical care. It is especially about how to accommodate those who do not now have medical insurance. These efforts are worthy endeavors, for sure, but I suggest that we first need to establish a vision for health care—determine what we really want—and then figure out how to pay for it. We are now putting the cart before the horse. Further, the cart is expensive and the horse needs some significant help if we are to have a truly healthy populace. The politicians and others who have engineered reform, in my opinion, also need to look at what is likely to transpire over the next five to fifteen years in medical care as a result of the rapid advances occurring in the biomedical, engineering, and computer sciences as described in my book *The Future of Medicine: Megatrends in Health Care That Will Improve Your Quality of Life*. These advances will materialize irrespective of reform and of whether the system is changed for the better. In addition, many other drivers of change will affect the delivery of medical care, including an aging population, a coming shortage of professionals, the rising consumerism, and the appalling changes in our behaviors that lead to preventable conditions such as obesity and stress. I will discuss these and other factors that are creating a major wave of change in how care is and will be delivered. We had better be prepared, or else reform may not be appropriate or helpful.

Still, the fundamental question is why has this change in the delivery system happened? Why do we tolerate a system that is a medical rather than a health-care system? Why do we accept a system that provides rather poor customer service and uneven or frankly inadequate results at prices that are simply unaffordable?

The answers are related to a payment system that is distorted, one in which the incentives to providers and patients alike are misaligned. True health-care reform needs to deal with these distortions, and concurrently we all need to accept certain responsibilities along with expected rights.

As individuals we have a responsibility to lead a reasonably healthy lifestyle. Our employers need to assist us with wellness programs. Insurers need to make it easier, not harder, to interact with them and to pay for appropriate care by our providers. Physicians need to realize that their practice patterns must become more patient centric (rather than provider centric), and they must give real attention to preventive care and thorough coordination of chronic illness care.

The government, for its part, needs to create incentives in the form of vouchers or tax credits for those who cannot obtain insurance; to develop a system to ensure that no one can go bankrupt as a result of illness; to encourage, not reduce, competition; and to create the necessary regulations to ensure the safety and efficacy of care, diagnostics, drugs, and devices. It must provide for public health in part through specific programs, but also through public education, taxes to discourage certain adverse health patterns, and incentives to encourage good health; through biomedical research; and through appropriate regulation (for example, food safety through the Food and Drug Administration [FDA] and the U.S. Department of Agriculture [USDA]) to assist in disease prevention and health promotion.

Incentives, rights, and responsibilities—each of these three elements are critical. They need to be appropriate and linked.

Let us begin with a look at the misconceptions of health-care delivery and health-care reform, and then review today's health-care system and why it does not work effectively. From this background, I will offer a vision for how an effective health-care delivery system should be organized. Then I will review where medical science is headed, followed by what changes, many of which will disrupt the current order, we can expect in hospital and outpatient care delivery in the coming years. Then I will turn to the issue of why medical care costs so much and why these costs are rising so rapidly. I will offer specific recommendations on how to bring these costs down in a manner that will actually lead to a much safer and better quality of care. This discussion will lead to a review of the recently passed health-care reform legislation. Finally, I will look at how our preferred system for future health care should be financed before summing up with what you can do personally *now* to have better health and spend less money.

2

What Really Needs to Change

Americans pride themselves on having a superior medical care system. We have superb medical schools, excellent hospital training programs, large numbers of nurses and pharmacists, the world's largest biomedical research endeavors that bring forth new methods of care, and the hub of the world's pharmaceutical and biotechnology industries. Further, we spend more for health care than any other country does on a per capita basis. Despite all of these advantages, our overall health is not the best, by far. By many measures, the United States ranks well below other countries. For example, infant mortality is higher and our life spans are shorter in the United States than they are in many other developed countries. Why are we left behind? As a country we focus on medical care for disease and injury, but four other important factors have as much, if not greater, impact on health: genetics, social circumstances, environmental exposures, and behavioral patterns. We can't change our genetics, and unfortunately social circumstances can often only be modified at the margin. Certainly we can do much better in dealing with the environmental issues. The single greatest opportunity to improve health and reduce premature deaths is in changing our personal behaviors. Our behaviors account for nearly 40 percent of all deaths in the United States.[1]

––––––– RANK ORDER OF CAUSES OF DEATH IN THE UNITED STATES
Tobacco use*
Poor diet/nutrition*
Lack of exercise*
Alcohol use to excess*
Infections

Toxic agents

Motor vehicle accidents*

Sexual behaviors*

Illicit drug use*

*Related to behavior

A. H. Mokdad et al., "Actual Causes of Death in the United States, 2000,"
Journal of American Medical Association 291, no. 10 (2004): 1238–45.

Here are some numbers to contemplate. In the United States, there are about 465,000 preventable deaths per year from smoking, 395,000 from high blood pressure, 216,000 from obesity, 191,000 from inactivity, 190,000 from high blood sugar levels, and 113,000 from high cholesterol. These causes of death are mostly, although not exclusively, related to our behaviors and lifestyles. The United States ranks thirty-ninth for infant mortality and thirty-sixth for life expectancy, yet we are first for per capita spending on health care.[2] Something is terribly wrong with this picture.

We cannot control many factors that affect our health. We cannot change our parents, many of us live in poverty where exposure to toxins such as lead paint is prevalent and food available for purchase is less than satisfactory, and many of us have less-than-adequate access to good health care. But among the factors that we can control and change are our behaviors. All too many Americans still smoke; many drink alcohol to excess and, more troubling, drive while intoxicated; and many do not wear seat belts. Although most of us have fluoridated water, many still have poor dental hygiene. We eat to excess and eat foods with little nutritional value, and we exercise all too little. We are on the verge of epidemics of diabetes, cardiovascular disease, and more because of these behaviors. It will not do to blame the fast-food industry, the soft drink manufacturers, or the cigarette or beer manufacturers without also taking personal responsibility for consuming their products. But we do need a national campaign to teach everyone what a healthy lifestyle is all about and educational programs to assist with smoking cessation, weight control, good nutrition, and stress management. We also need meaningful monetary incentives in the form of insurance premium reductions to help us change our behaviors. Our medical care system is poorly designed to deal with this crisis and certainly is not incentivized to tackle it. Generalist physicians are not paid to spend time with patients to teach them about diet and exercise or the benefits of not smoking. Nor is anyone else paid to do it! We need a political initiative to address the issues and changes in compensation for health-care professionals that in turn will allow them to assist patients in ways that will have a major impact on health into the future. For example, primary care physicians need to be incentivized to spend time on preventive medicine (for example, counseling for tobacco cessation, nutrition, weight loss, and exercise) and to coordinate the care of their patients with chronic illnesses who must visit many specialists and undergo many diagnostic tests or procedures. Both efforts would markedly improve the quality of care, improve patients' health, and reduce expenditures. The goal is all about adjusting the financial incentives for both providers and the population at large.

We need to appreciate how diseases have changed dramatically over the past century, and we must change our approaches to deal with the diseases that are now rampant. At the beginning of the twentieth century when my grandfather started his medical practice, the most common causes of death were pneumonia and tuberculosis, both of which are far down the list today. Indeed, for most of human history, infectious diseases and malnutrition were the major reasons why the average expectancy was only about thirty years. Then with the industrial age came sanitation, the first vaccines, and better nutrition, with a consequent decline in infant mortality and a rise in life expectancy. But then, smoking and dietary changes led to more cardiovascular diseases and cancers by the mid-twentieth century and beyond. Now, although smoking has declined, obesity and lack of exercise have led to rapid increases in diabetes, heart disease, stroke, and high blood pressure plus joint disease, cancers, sleep apnea, asthma, and many other chronic illnesses that last a lifetime.[3]

Unless and until we as a society deal with our behaviors, our health status will not improve. Yes, access to medical care is important, and it is beyond belief that our country does not afford everyone easy and affordable access to medical care. As a society we also need to offer everyone a good education so that they can be productive and increase their standard of living. Our insistence on a diet high in fat and sugar, our lack of exercise, our persistent use of tobacco, and our unwillingness to do the simple things in life such as brush our teeth, however, will condemn many of us to a life of poor or at least inadequate health. We individuals need incentives to change our habits and behaviors. A reduction in health insurance premiums for either engaging in good behaviors or taking action to lose weight, stop smoking, and start exercising would be a positive incentive.

As to medical care, our quality is fairly good, although it is certainly not as good as it could or should be. The problem is twofold. First, our medical care system does not deal with health; it concentrates on illness, or "disease and pestilence." Second, we poorly manage the more complex illnesses that are chronic, such as diabetes, heart failure, and cancer.

According to a report for the World Economic Forum released in September 2011,

> Non-communicable diseases have been established as a clear threat not only to human health, but also to development and economic growth. Claiming 63% of all deaths, these diseases are currently the world's main killer. Eighty percent of these deaths now occur in low- and middle-income countries. Half of those who die of chronic non-communicable diseases are in the prime of their productive years, and thus, the disability imposed and the lives lost are also endangering industry competitiveness across borders.[4]

These chronic illnesses have become much more common and consume a huge amount of the total cost of health care. The Milken Institute quantified some of these issues in a research report a few years ago. They evaluated cancer, diabetes, hypertension, stroke, heart disease, pulmonary conditions, and mental disorders. Here are some of the key findings:

> More than 109 million Americans report having at least one of the seven diseases, for a total of 162 million cases. The total impact of these diseases on the economy is $1.3 trillion annually. On our current path, in 2023 we project a 42 percent increase in cases of the seven chronic diseases and $4.2 trillion in treatment costs and lost economic output. Lower obesity rates alone could produce productivity gains of $254 billion and avoid $60 billion in treatment expenditures per year.[5]

To me the important point is that "each has been linked to behavioral and/or environmental risk factors that broad-based prevention programs could address."[6]

The fundamental problem is that our delivery system was designed to deal with acute problems, not chronic ones. A single physician can treat most acute illnesses such as an ear infection. Chronic illnesses, however, require a team approach with well-coordinated care to ensure quality outcomes, safe care, and reasonable or at least not excessive costs. Indeed, good care coordination can reduce the number of doctor visits, procedures, tests, and even hospitalizations required, resulting in better care for less cost. But we do not have this setup today.

Instead, our system is a medical care system, not a health-care system. Further, good care is only good if a person can access it, and we clearly lack in access given that 47 million Americans are without insurance and many more are underinsured. America is the only country in the developed world that does not ensure all its citizens will have access to basic medical care and that their catastrophic needs will be covered. The current reform bill, the Patient Protection and Affordable Care Act, will add about 31 million to the insurance rolls, so it will make a big dent in the problem. Add the paucity of general or primary care physicians in the inner cities and rural areas, however, and it becomes apparent that access to care by those who most need it is deficient, whether or not they have insurance. Those without insurance or ready access to a provider or both have worse health, and ultimately their poor health status increases all of our costs when these individuals end up in the ER with a major problem that could have and should have been treated simply and cheaply much earlier.

Further, most of us find that we get too little time with our physician when we do have an office visit, and we leave feeling that we were not listened to, not understood, and not certain whether the plan of care was really the best it could be. Add to all of this tension the frustration of dealing with the insurance companies, the paperwork, the phone calls, the time to get an appointment, and the lack of coordinated care among providers, and it is no wonder that medical care is nowhere near what it could be and not what it should be, especially given that 17 percent of our gross domestic product (GDP) is committed to health care.

This 17 percent of the GDP is double what it was thirty years ago and is expected to reach 20 percent during the next decade. This increase stems from costs rising at about 6–10 percent per year, or well above the country's general rate of inflation. Clearly this rate of increase cannot continue indefinitely. It is negatively affecting businesses' profitability and, indeed, their survivability, and it means that raises in wage are limited because the money available is going for health insurance. Most workers do not appreciate this fact. The government cannot continue to pay more since there is a limit to how much it can tax to cover the costs. As individuals, we already are saddled with high insurance premiums, co-pays, and deductibles and are frustrated to say the least. All of this information suggests that the first place to start with health-care reform is to decide what our system of care should be, then address the way to improve quality while reducing costs of care, and finally tackle access issues. That process will be my recommendation throughout this book.

Medicare and Medicaid together represent about half of all medical care spending in the United States. As this outlay increases it will become a burden that the federal and state governments cannot sustain any more than General Motors could. General Motors passed retiree health-care costs off to the unions, but the country cannot foist them off to any other entity. As the population ages and the numbers of elderly increase, federal cost hikes will not slow and certainly will not drop. Peter Orszag, the former director of the Congressional Budget Office (CBO), a nonpartisan agency of Congress, has stated that "our country's financial health will in fact be determined primarily by the growth rate of per capita healthcare costs." Yet discussions of Medicare and Medicaid policy as well as of broader health-care reforms have not seriously addressed the issue of how to slow growth in spending.[7] To date the government's only real effort to reduce Medicare costs has been to cap payments to physicians and hospitals. But limiting remuneration is not a strategy. In fact, it tends to worsen the overall problem because it further shifts costs to others. Physicians and hospitals need to be part of the solution, but they cannot control the myriad elements of the health-care system that need to be brought together to effect real and lasting reductions in costs. But as I will explain later, there is much that they can and should do right now to lower the costs of care.

With such high costs it would seem logical that we Americans should have the best medical care and even the best health care overall. Indeed, many will argue that in fact our care is the best in the world. But unfortunately it is simply not true; the data does not support that contention. We have a long way to go to reach our full potential. With rapidly rising costs, it would seem that we could easily enough identify the causes and then address them with American ingenuity, but we seem to focus on the wrong issues or simply avoid the issues that are more difficult to address. So I will wade into this morass and try to explain why costs are rising and what needs to be done to bring them down while at the same time improving our overall health status.

THE CRITICAL ISSUES CONFRONTING HEALTH-CARE
DELIVERY AND HEALTH-CARE REFORM

The following are the major delivery issues confronting our system today. Any effective reform package needs to address these issues in order for it to have a really helpful and cost-neutral impact that is satisfying to patients and providers alike.

Delivery Recommendations

- Shift the delivery model to focus on complex, chronic illnesses.
- Establish good care coordination for those with chronic illness and catastrophic disease or injury.
- Encourage more physicians to enter primary care (and certain specialties such as general surgery).
- Offer sound preventive care and wellness management.
- Shift from the diagnose-and-treat paradigm to one of prediction and prevention.
- Focus on safety and equality.

Reform Recommendations

- Access—ensure quality health care for all regardless of ability to pay by giving them insurance and ensuring that providers are available.
- Insurance—set mandates, community ratings, preexisting conditions, and premium variations based on behaviors, such as smoking, weight, and exercise. Individuals to own policy with high deductibles.
- Payments—reconsider how physicians, hospitals, and other providers receive payment, that is, per a visit or procedure or via capitation or by bundling with measures of quality and safety.
- Delivery—reorganize how medicine is delivered to each of us (intimately tied to payment reform).
- Costs—reduce as a result of the preceding reforms if properly implemented.

THE MISCONCEPTIONS ABOUT HEALTH-CARE DELIVERY
AND HEALTH-CARE REFORM

A group of misconceptions surrounds the current efforts to discuss health-care reform. I am puzzled that political leaders, media commentators, and others are not addressing all of the issues and frequently are missing the most important issues. Reform, as it has been debated in Congress, will deal with some elements of the issues and problems besetting health care, but it ignores many others. The problem is, these matters are critical. If only some of the issues are addressed, the result will be a major escalation of costs, taxes, and greater frustration. Today it is extremely important at least to put all the issues out for discussion and then let the political and other processes begin to address them. Decision makers probably will not tackle them all at once, but at least they should recognize that all of them must be addressed in the not-too-distant future.

Misconception 1. *America has the best health care in the world.*

Sorry, but again this assertion is not true. As stated before, we have a medical care system, not a health-care system. We do spend more per capita than any other country does on health care, but our quality of care does not measure up to what we spend. The United States has a higher infant mortality rate (6.9 deaths per 1,000 live births) than do many countries (Japan, 2.8; France, 3.9); and our life span (77.9 years) has not kept up (Japan, 83; Switzerland, 82). We have lifesaving vaccines available, but nearly 20 percent of American infants do not receive them. Only about one-third of us are at a healthy weight. About 20 percent of us still smoke. Regular exams are not sought regularly, and screenings for preventable or reversible problems such as high blood pressure, high cholesterol, and cancer are all too often not obtained. In short, the American health-care system responds, and responds fairly well, to illness and trauma, but as these numbers document, it is not focused on preventive medicine. Further, we do not have coordinated care for those with complex, chronic diseases like heart failure and cancer. These diseases cannot be treated appropriately with our current helter-skelter approach in which independent physicians refer patients to each other as the situation warrants instead of following a well-coordinated system for addressing all of the patients' needs in an organized manner with multidisciplinary teams.

Misconception 2. *Health-care reform will have an impact on the advances in medical science.*

No. Health-care reform is not about scientific advances; instead, it is about insurance and how to pay for it. We have a robust set of programs in the United States that are advancing science and are funded by the National Institutes of Health, the pharmaceutical industry, and the biotechnology and medical devices industries. These programs will not change with reform.

Misconception 3. *Health-care reform will improve the delivery of care and offer us better care opportunities.*

In fact, health-care reform addresses mostly the ways to pay for medical care for the uninsured and only somewhat the rising costs of medical care. I use the term "medical care" here to emphasize that today American health care focuses mainly on treating disease and injury and little on promoting wellness and preventing illness. While the reforms address the financing of medical care, they ignore the quality and the safety of health care and, given the coming shortages of professionals at all levels, who will deliver it and how. Certainly it is important to ensure access to care for everyone, but don't let that issue confuse you into thinking your health-care delivery will be improved. It will not.

Misconception 4. *The remarkable advances from the basic biological, engineering, and computer sciences are rapidly made available to the medical care delivery system and to the patients who can most benefit from them.*
We should hope this assertion is true, but often it is simply not the case. Some new technologies of great value are slow to be adopted, such as using simulation for teaching procedures rather than learning by practicing on the patient. Sometimes delays occur because people are reluctant to abandon the old way, or "the way we have always done it," and sometimes because those who control the finances do not appreciate the new developments' underlying value.

Misconception 5. *Health-care costs will be reduced if we have an electronic medical record.*
No doubt establishing an electronic medical record (EMR) will be valuable for patient care quality and safety, but it will be difficult to implement until and unless the available systems include a good process for physicians to document patient care— that is, history, physical examination, and clinical progress notes. Further, standards must be established to allow for interoperability among competing systems so that records can be shared when appropriate from caregiver to caregiver. Creating a mandate or a financial incentive for every practitioner to use an EMR will not be enough and not by a long shot. In fact, as with promoting increased access and coverage, mandating an EMR, even with the government helping to pay for it, will substantially drive up costs before it ever assists in reducing them.

Misconception 6. *Universal coverage for all Americans will reduce costs.*
Unfortunately universal coverage instead will create substantial added expenditures. America is the only country in the developed world that does not have some system to ensure everyone has at least basic medical care coverage. Shame on us. But offering coverage to all will cost someone—namely, you and me—in taxes. Certainly it is true that guaranteeing access to a physician for basic medical care will mean fewer visits to the ER, fewer hospitalizations, and better overall health for the individual. It will

reduce the cost of care, but there are still substantial real costs for providing medical care to 31 million additional people. To think otherwise is to ignore reality.

Misconception 7. *Health-care costs are rising because of the avarice and greed of unregulated "bad guys," including drug and technology companies, doctors, hospitals, malpractice lawyers, and third-party payers, or insurers.*

Each of these groups deserves some approbation and bears some responsibility at the margin, but they are not the major reasons why costs are rising. But it seems that politicians, the media, and so many others seem to believe what's convenient rather than what is accurate. As *Fortune* magazine editor Allan Sloan once observed, "It is the whale that comes to the surface that gets harpooned."[8]

The real culprits for health care's rising costs are:

1. The poor coordination of care of those with chronic illness resulting in excess visits to specialists, more tests, unneeded procedures, and even hospitalizations.

2. The overuse (often as a result of the first culprit) of expensive drugs, devices, or procedures when they are not needed or truly necessary or when a generic drug, older device, or no procedure at all would be more than adequate and appropriate.

3. A wide divergence in the use of medical care and technologies based on geographic region with no evidence that those who receive more resources have better health outcomes or longer lives.

4. An aging population that gets sick more often and consumes more medical care.

5. Physicians, patients, or relatives who are unwilling to accept the inevitability of death and insist on "one last try."

6. Preventable errors that lead to at least 100,000 people dying annually of safety lapses (from a hospital-acquired infection or drug or procedural mistakes), and many more being harmed.

7. Over time, our own behaviors along with a lack of preventive medicine or wellness programs.

Misconception 8. *New technologies are major culprits in rising health-care costs.*

Advancements present a double-edged sword. New technologies can be lifesaving and life enhancing and actually reduce total costs of care, but if used inappropriately, they can result in more costs. It is true that many technologies, such as drugs, devices, imaging, procedures, and so on, are used unnecessarily. Mostly this nonessential treatment occurs with those patients who have chronic illnesses. Many do not benefit from good care coordination by their physicians and hence end up with too many unneeded visits to specialists, too many tests, and duplication of medications.

Misconception 9. *If my doctor prescribes a drug, orders a test, or suggests a medical device, I should go with that recommendation.*

It is a good idea to discuss each recommendation; do not accept advice blindly. Is the drug really necessary and what are its potential side effects? Is a generic equivalent available? Is a similar drug that costs less available? Will the test result actually guide the therapy, or is it merely being done to have a "complete" record of care? Has the device been proven to be useful for my situation? What is the evidence? And in every case, always ask about the added costs. Remember your body and your health are important, and you should be satisfied that your care is indeed appropriate.

Misconception 10. *Comparative effectiveness research is nothing but a government method to begin care rationing.*

Medicine needs to know what works and what does not. Many professional societies do their best to bring together the available information, but much more needs to be accomplished toward that end. We need more well-done scientific evaluations and better distribution of that information to the provider community—and to patients, for that matter.

Misconception 11. *We need to have many systems in place to detect fraud and abuse. Without them, costs would skyrocket even further.*

Medical care consumes vast amounts of money. On the one hand, it is no surprise that the unscrupulous will try to take advantage with fraud and abuse. On the other hand, loads of administrative waste already exist in the medical system. Get rid of it, and costs will plummet. Insurers use their high overheads to service their claims and search for fraud and errors in billed claims. Indeed, they employ a workforce that equals half of the number of practicing physicians. Hospitals also have immense staffs to bill insurers and patients and to check if a patient has stayed too long in the hospital. Physicians need large staffs to deal with insurers and to obtain permission for their patients to get a computed tomography (CT) scan or to refer them to a specialist. All of this effort represents essentially wasted money in that it is not being used to care for patients. Any part of a real reform should, and indeed must, cut this waste. It will save real money and, more important, get everyone in the health-care field back to doing useful work and improving the lives of their patients.

Misconception 12. *Safety is a problem of poor care but is not a significant cost issue.*
As noted in misconception 7, more than 100,000 individuals die of preventable medical errors each year and untold more have serious but not fatal outcomes. Not only can an error do harm, but it also can lead to big cost increases. For example, a hospital-acquired infection can add days to the patient's stay and require an expensive antibiotic, which in turn may have side effects and perhaps require time in an ICU. If your pharmacy gives you the wrong medication, it can result in an expensive hospitalization. If the staff pays inadequate attention to discharge instructions, it may lead to the patient's unplanned and unexpected return to the hospital or the ER. All of these expensive and preventable errors are major drivers of the high cost of medical care.

Misconception 13. *As with other elements of the marketplace, giving patients more control of their health-care expenditures will lead to lower costs.*
It makes good sense for all of us to become more involved in our health-care decision making and in its payments. But individuals "buy" health care differently than they do any other purchase. Patients or their loved ones do not shop for the best price the way they shop for a new washing machine. They look for the best (as they understand it) physician, hospital, and so on. Mostly they accept their personal physician's advice regarding drugs, surgery, or rehabilitation. That said, it makes sense to have high-deductible policies with or without health savings accounts (HSAs) or medical savings accounts (MSAs) that will encourage each of us to examine each "purchase" our physician recommends and often will lead to less expensive alternatives. These policies, along with HSAs and MSAs, give individuals the opportunity to obtain care with pretax dollars, a nice savings, and bring insurance back to its true purpose— that is, coverage for catastrophic expenses and not prepaid total health care as is most insurance today.

The more we know about our medical care costs and the more we ask our providers why a test, a drug, or a procedure is necessary then the more likely we will see a reduction in total costs. Being more directly invested in the costs of our care will ultimately have this market effect. Unfortunately, as patients we still have an information gap relative to our provider. We need to stop accepting advice without questioning, and being directly responsible for how our health-care dollars are spent might provoke that change.

Misconception 14. *The insurance companies are the primary culprits causing insurance premiums to rise.*
It is easy to castigate the insurers, but to a large degree they are simply the middlemen in this whole broken process. Their role is to assess how much care will cost for a group of people—say, employees in a large company—and then collect that money and pay it out over the year to the various providers. The insurer is not the cause of rising medical costs; instead, it is the system in place, which we all seem to tolerate, albeit grumpily.

Misconception 15. *Primary care physicians do not deal with the expensive aspects of medical care so they can have little impact on reducing medical expenditures.*
Two major reasons for cost escalation are the lack of good care coordination of those with complex, chronic illnesses and inadequate attention to prevention and screening. PCPs are key to changing both of these issues, but they are allotted too little time per patient and are not paid for either activity (the latter will change somewhat with the new reform legislation). About 5 percent of all health-care expenditures go to PCPs, but they can have a major impact on how the other 95 percent is spent, especially with good care coordination of chronic illness and with a focus on prevention. To fix this situation, PCPs need to be incentivized, or paid, to deliver care coordination for the chronically ill and good preventive care to all of their patients. This investment could see a high return and have a huge impact on total costs. It is a logical place to begin to address the high costs of medical care in America.

Misconception 16. *New technologies increase costs, reduce productivity, and have little beneficial effect on safety and quality care.*
Of course, it is not the new technology per se that is at fault for rising costs. It is the improper or excessive use of a test, device, drug, or procedure that drives up costs. The technology, when used properly, may well save patients' lives or improve their health. And some technologies can actually reduce costs by improving quality, safety, and provider productivity.

Misconception 17. *Health-care reform will offer access to all, or nearly all, while reducing the costs of care.*

Giving about 31 million of the currently 47 million uninsured individuals medical care insurance will markedly increase expenditures. It is true that if these individuals get appropriate care at the right time with vaccines, screenings, preventive care, and annual exams then some diseases will be prevented and others such as high blood pressure will be detected before they cause serious harm. But today in the United States we spend about $7,500 annually per person on medical care. Adding more people to the rolls will certainly increase costs.

Misconception 18. *Health-care reform will fundamentally improve how we receive care going forward.*

This development is also not at all likely except for those who now do not have medical care insurance. For the rest of us, medical care delivery will only change because of fundamental societal and demographic reasons along with the marked difference in the types, severity, and chronicity of illnesses that is occurring right now. What reform may do is offer patients with a preexisting condition the ability to purchase insurance and at a reasonable premium cost.

Misconception 19. *Health care is or should be a right, not a privilege and not a responsibility.*

During the 2008 presidential debates, Tom Brokaw asked, "Is health care a right, a privilege, or a responsibility?" The candidates did not answer the question, but now Congress and Barack Obama's administration should balance the rights being offered as part of health-care reform with the corresponding responsibilities.

Congress rightly seeks to ensure access to care for all people regardless of their ability to pay. It is appropriate then for the taxpayer to expect the recipients in return to lead a reasonably healthy lifestyle, not only to maintain and improve their health, but also to cut the cost of their care. Congress also is banning the insurers' practice of excluding individuals with predisposing conditions. A reasonable expectation, or responsibility, in return is that everyone will participate in insurance and keep the risk pool large and the costs down; but this hotly debated issue is now in the courts. In another pairing of rights with responsibilities, commercial insurers and Medicare should be able to incentivize patients to hold down costs by offering premium reductions for those who take care of their health. This combination of rights and responsibilities satisfies the legitimate arguments of those who insist that medical care is a right with the equally important argument that we all must accept a meaningful level of responsibility for our health and its costs.

Misconception 20. *The only health-care reform that matters is what the federal government implements; providers and employers can do little.*
Actually everyone can do a great deal now toward reform. Insurers can create incentives for care coordination and prevention, industry can develop wellness programs, providers can attend to care coordination and prevention, and all of us can take responsibility for maintaining our own health.

Misconception 21. *If waste in medical care is eliminated or at least markedly curtailed, there will not be a need to limit what insurance covers.*
Sorry, but it ultimately will be necessary to limit what insurance covers; otherwise, the costs of care become prohibitive. Either we have less generous benefits or some people will be without coverage. Call it rationing if you must, but the better term might be "rational."

Misconception 22. *"I cannot do very much to prevent disease as I get older; it all depends on my doctor or what is in my genes."*
Your doctor can and will assist with the detection and treatment of disease and can offer you vaccines, preventive measures, and screening tests. Your genes certainly are important. But you can do a great deal to live a good life: eat well, exercise regularly, manage stress, and not smoke. You can brush and floss well, use your seat belts, and not drive while drinking, talking on the phone, texting, or eating. You will be healthier, feel better, live longer, and spend less money.

3

What Change Looks Like: A Vision for the Future

Misconception: *America has the best health care in the world.*

Howard County, Maryland, is located between Baltimore and Washington, D.C. Largely rural farmland until 1965, it is now home to Columbia, the planned community inspired by James Rouse, and a rapidly growing population. The schools are considered excellent, the library has been voted among the best in the nation, and the median income is among the nation's highest. Still, some people there are without insurance. Some are indigent; some, who consider themselves young and invincible, choose not to purchase insurance; and some are employed by businesses, primarily service industries, that do not offer insurance. Some can afford it but choose to spend their income on other needs. The county has many primary care physicians, although many PCPs are not taking new patients. There are excellent specialists available, the community hospital is highly regarded, and highly recognized academic medical centers are nearby in Baltimore and Washington for tertiary care needs. In short, medical care in Howard County is very good, yet an estimated twenty thousand individuals do not have health insurance.

County Executive Ken Ulman and the health officer, Dr. Peter Beilenson, with a master's degree in public health (MPH), were determined to establish a model program based on the dual concept that everyone would have basic health care but that each person must take responsibility for his or her health as a prerequisite for participation. They created the Healthy Howard, a community-supported, not-for-profit network into which members pay a nominal fee. They have access to a PCP group practice for unlimited visits. A pharmacy benefits manager, employed by Healthy Howard, is located at the PCP offices and helps members find the most cost-conscious choice of prescription. A care coordinator is also located at the PCP offices and works with patients to manage complex care plans. Specialists in the county have agreed to see referred patients on a pro bono basis, assured that none of them will have to take a disproportionate share. The local hospital, which always took patients who could not afford to pay, will not bill members of the plan at all. Since the hospital is part of the Johns Hopkins Health System, Hopkins' hospital also has agreed to accept at no charge those patients who need tertiary hospitalization. And the entire program is all tied together with a simple electronic medical record.

The other part of the plan is that each member has a health coach. Together the coach and the member develop a strategy for healthy living in conjunction with the care plan of the member's PCP. It might include a program to stop smoking, to start exercising, or to lose weight. The member meets with the coach regularly to check compliance and progress. The coach helps if there is a barrier. For example, if a grandmother cannot go to the local gym for exercise because she babysits her grandchild while her single daughter works, the coach will try to find a day care arrangement and a gym that will take her either pro bono or at a reduced rate. So the plan tries to help members overcome obstacles while still expecting them to meet their personal responsibility for healthy living.

The hope is that members' overall health will improve while good primary care will reduce the costs of care, including the need for specialists, emergency room visits, and hospitalizations. The plan's founders recognize that initially at least the plan may detect previously undiagnosed or untreated problems, such as hypertension or high cholesterol, that will increase current costs, yet in the long term intervention will improve health and reduce total expenditures. They have contracted with schools of public health to do unbiased analyses over time of the program's efficacy and its economic results.

The plan's fundamental vision is "rights with responsibility." It is not true insurance, but it does offer basic medical and preventive services at a nominal cost while mobilizing the best of the medical care community to assist. Time will tell how well it works, but there is every reason to be optimistic. The plan ensures everyone receives good care while they work to overcome the barriers to healthy living. It represents a real vision for health care into the future.

The first key step in any set of decisions about the future of health care is to envision the care system, *then* the payment system. Most efforts to date begin with the payment system and ignore the care system.

Politicians and pundits are concerned, rightly, about those people without insurance coverage, and everyone is worried about costs. But few ever focus on the system of actual care. In efforts to reform the system, it is absolutely critical that we first define the desired system of care and then, and only then, address how to pay for it and how to keep the costs down. Knowing what type of care system we want will lead us to design a financing structure that, in turn, will allow us to create the incentives to achieve the desired system of care. Whatever the vision of health care for the future, it will need to be paid for, so the plan realistically must include methods to slow the rise of health-care costs. Without this critical step, there will be no funds left to improve the system.

We have to decide if our current care delivery system is appropriate and adequate. Do we want this system, or do we want and need something else, something better? To develop a better system we will need to fund creativity, not destroy it. While I have a preference for a private, market-driven system rather than a government-organized system, whatever we develop needs to allow for creativity and to produce real incentives to drive the necessary end points. Too much regulation, too many mandates, and too many policies—no matter their good intent—ultimately will prevent a good outcome. Likewise, by establishing too few regulations or the wrong regulations, the system will become uncontrolled and focused on profits, on processes, or on forms instead of care.

A VISION FOR TRUE HEALTH CARE

With that discussion in mind and based on more than 150 extensive interviews with health-care leaders from across the country such as hospital CEOs and COOs, academic and practicing physicians, pharmacists, insurance industry managers, and many others, here are some thoughts as to what a vision for health care might entail. First, there is a crucial need for more prevention, wellness, and health promotion efforts. We fall way short in this regard today, so it will mean a combination of public and private activities through the Centers for Disease Control, the Food and Drug Administration, and the Department of Agriculture on the federal level. It will mean much more attention in our schools to exercise, healthy foods, and basic health education. And it will mean personal attention to health promotion and disease prevention activities by each of us as individuals. The system also should include incentives for all of us to maintain our health as best we can, given what is already known about promoting wellness and preventing illness. It must also improve the coordination of complex disease management among the myriad providers. We need rapid, easy access to primary care providers; they have been and should continue to be the backbone of the health-care delivery system in America. A shortage of primary care physicians exists now and likely will be exacerbated in the coming years, so we must take steps to encourage medical school graduates to enter primary care fields. Further, the PCPs need to have more time with their patients, and that stipulation means increasing their reimbursements for their time spent dealing with prevention and wellness as well as coordinating chronic illness care.

Some of us simply will not be able to afford insurance, and given the wealth of our country, it is incomprehensible that we have not found a way to guarantee catastrophic coverage and basic preventive care for those who are truly in need. For everyone else, we need a simplified financing system and a return to true insurance with large risk pools. The perverse incentives to order more tests, do more procedures, prescribe more medications, and refer to more specialists—all of which drive up costs—need to be addressed. As part of this change, patients and doctors need to return to a contractual relationship akin to other professional service arrangements. Insurance by its very definition should be for catastrophic needs, allowing each of us as individuals to take personal responsibility through high deductibles to pay for routine care. The hurdles (which I will discuss in chapter 12) that doctors, hospitals, and patients all face now with their insurance companies need to be eliminated. Another critical aspect of the financing of health care is that for its programs, the government must pay its fair share of the cost. Today it definitely does not. Finally, our vision of health care for the future must include immediate access—that is, available anytime and anyplace—to digitized yet secure medical information.

Let's take a closer look at what we have today. The current system of care focuses on acute medical care. It is a disease-oriented system and certainly not a health management or patient-oriented system. Mostly, this situation arose owing to a reimbursement methodology extending back to the 1950s or so that underrates the medical generalists and tilts toward those who do procedures. That focus is not what we need; instead, we need a payment system that rewards the generalist for working in rural or socio-economically deprived areas, for taking the time to listen to the patient, and for being attuned to prevention and wellness management. Today in America we need to change the system to focus on disease prevention and health promotion, with ready access to primary care and its providers. Then, when necessary, it should grant access to specialists, hospitals, rehabilitation, and all the other requirements for good medical care when disease or injury does occur. (I should note that this arrangement does work fairly well in some staff model health maintenance organizations [HMOs] such as Kaiser Permanente, where a capitation system encourages the physicians to provide preventive medicine along with care coordination of chronic illnesses, not only diagnosis and treatment.)

In addition, our medical care system has developed around diagnosing and treating acute illnesses such as pneumonia, a gall bladder attack, or appendicitis. In these cases, the internist prescribes an antibiotic and the surgeon removes the gall bladder or the appendix, and the patient is cured. But as the population ages, more and more individuals are developing complex, chronic diseases such as heart failure, diabetes, lung disease, or cancer. These diseases remain with the individual for life and require a different approach to care. Instead of episodic care, these patients need long-term care in which one physician serves as the orchestrator and manages the myriad physician specialists and the other caregivers for a unified, team-based approach. Chronic diseases are expensive to treat; indeed, heart disease and diabetes alone account for more than half of health-care costs in America. We need a new approach to managing these patients, both to improve their care and to reduce the costs. The new approach actually already exists in some locations; we need to understand what works and then replicate it nationally. More than anything else, the PCP still must coordinate patient care and ensure top quality at a reasonable cost.

LEVERAGING TECHNOLOGY

Concurrently, we need to exploit technology, especially information technology. Again, however, our payment system is a disincentive. Physicians do not get paid for e-mail encounters, telephone consults with patients, or telemedicine activities. We have the technology to route information and improve and maximize skills, but the hurdle is that insurance, both government and commercial, limits payments to conducting an in-person diagnostic or treatment visit rather than for preventing a disease or coordinating the care of chronic illnesses.

INCENTIVES FOR PATIENTS AND PROVIDERS

We need a system that incentivizes both patients to stay well and doctors to help their patients stay well. Today insurance pays at the *margin* but not at the *core* of this issue. The system should pay providers for actually providing health care in addition to improving payments for comprehensive disease care, instead of for a single visit or for a procedure. Insurers generally do not want to spend money on a patient's preventive care because they see it as a current cost for a possible savings later, and they might not accrue that savings because the person might not be insured with their company in the future. It is a catch-22.

INSURANCE: BACK TO BASICS

Personally, I believe we need to revert to the insurance system where we each paid out of pocket for basic care and used insurance for the large, unexpected, or catastrophic events.[1] Today, what we call insurance actually has morphed into prepaid care, meaning that we use our insurance to pay for everything, including annual visits, basic medications, and all sorts of important but routine care. This shift also means since someone else—for example, an employer or the government—is paying most of the insurance bill that we are no longer contracting directly with our provider, so we do not know what the total costs are. Instead, why not pay for basic medical expenses out of pocket and save our insurance for what it was always intended to cover, namely, unexpected high-cost events. In the case of medical care, it would provide surgery, procedures, hospitalizations, and expensive medicines such as those for cancer. For those unfortunate enough to develop a complex, chronic illness (or illnesses), it would be for the myriad doctors, tests, procedures, and drugs needed. If it was used in this manner, medical care insurance would be much less expensive, and many more could afford it. (I will explain the rationale for this concept in more detail in chapters 12 and 16.)

Here is a look at the increase in health-care costs over the past decades. The per capita expenditures have risen from $356 in 1970, to $1,091 in 1980, to $2,810 in 1990, to $4,703 in 2000, and by 2008 had reached $7,538.[2] In the 1970s we mostly paid out of pocket, except for "catastrophic" needs that were covered by relatively low-cost insurance. Today, we essentially purchase "prepaid" health care and have limited reason to focus our attention on the total dollar amount. It is time to get back to a system where we connect with the provider in a typical professional relationship.

PROVIDERS

One of the key choke points in reform may well be the physician, or specifically the number of practicing physicians in the future, what their specialties are, and where they are located. There are too few physicians now, and the shortage will grow as most residents choose to enter a specialty rather than become general internists, general pediatricians, or family physicians. Frankly, money is the issue. Generalists are underpaid and paid even more poorly in rural or socio-economically deprived areas where the major insurer is often Medicaid. They need incentives, not disincentives, to provide good preventive care and equally good chronic illness care. In addition, we will need new kinds of health-care professionals who can assist the generalist, along with more and better use of nurse practitioners (NPs), physician assistants, optometrists, pharmacists, physical therapists, social workers, and other care providers. Physicians, especially generalists, need to accept these practitioners rather than, as all too often happens today, trying to marginalize them. The idea is not to replace the generalist, but to enhance his or her productivity so that the generalist can provide really complete primary health care.

PATIENTS FIRST

Of course, to be a care system that we can all appreciate, it must always put the patient and the patient's family first. Throughout the new health-care system, patients must be regarded as customers and hence respected because they are contracting (paying) with the provider (doctor, hospital, ER, etc.) for the service. It must be understood that they will expect prompt, courteous, and professional service and care that is based on the most recent evidence-based information available. Likewise, the insurance companies need to regard the individual as the customer, not an annoyance.

Today the insurer sees the government or employers as their customers, not the patient. Doctors, in turn, see the insurer as their source of payment, not the patient. So the patient is no one's customer and is treated accordingly. Thus, the incentives for the patient's treatment are seriously misaligned.

Information should be readily forthcoming, and the insurers' forms should be comprehensive yet easy to read. Our medical records need to be considered ours, not belonging to the physician or the hospital, and we should have access to them at any time or place. With access, we can read them and request a factual error be changed. Of course, patients should receive care of the highest quality and feel safe from preventable errors and harm. This expectation should not be too much to ask. Indeed, it will be up to each of us to insist on this level of and approach to care, and if we do not get it, we should feel perfectly free and empowered to go elsewhere, taking our medical information with us in a convenient digital format.

PUBLIC HEALTH

America has an incredible research engine fueled by the National Institutes of Health, our medical schools, the pharmaceutical industry, the biotechnology industry, and the medical device industry. But all of these organizations and agencies are largely focused on curing disease and not on maintaining good health. The true health needs of the nation and the world are public health questions. Here we spend all too little; indeed, the anthrax incidents in 2001 and Hurricane Katrina in 2005 proved that we are ill prepared to deal with public health problems. Some government and church leaders refuse to acknowledge how HIV-AIDS is spread and instead prevent agencies from distributing condoms. Food-borne illnesses have become epidemic. We allow antibiotics to be used in poultry and cattle and then wonder about the spread of antibiotic-resistant bacteria from hamburger or chicken to humans. The Department of Agriculture stamps the fattiest beef as "prime," and we subsidize the production of corn to produce high-fructose corn syrup for everything from sodas to candy. We have slowly but surely changed from a country that produces nutritious food to one that manufactures commodity products of low nutritional value.

New York City is trying to address some of these issues. Former longtime commissioner of health (and now director of the CDC) Thomas Freiden addressed key public health issues with support from Mayor Michael Bloomberg (the mayor served as chairman of the board of Johns Hopkins University and gave an endowment of $100 million to the School of Public Health, which now bears his name). Sodas are no longer available in city schools. Trans fats have been banned in fast-food restaurants. Similar to how the health department handles cases of tuberculosis, every time a diabetic patient undergoes a test called Hemoglobin A1c, which measures the stability of blood sugar levels, it is filed with the health department so that it can follow up the report. The idea is to ensure the diabetic patient is getting the care he or she needs since it will prevent untold major and enormously costly problems later in life.

Other approaches to public health would be banning smoking in public places, taxing cigarettes, seeking voluntary (on the part of manufacturers) reductions in salt and sugar in foods and sodas, and taxing sugar in sodas. Public education, such as First Lady Michelle Obama's campaign to raise awareness about good eating habits (starting in childhood) along with vigorous exercise, is an absolutely critical aspect of public health.

The Institute of Medicine in its 2003 publication *Who Will Keep the Public Healthy?* concludes "we are facing problems no one has seen before."[3] Lifestyle-related diseases, such as obesity-induced type 2 diabetes in children, will place a new toll on health care and health-care providers. Recognizing that many, indeed most, of the causes of illness and premature death are preventable, public health now and in the future must address individual lifestyles, living and working environments, education, cultural factors, and government policies.

It is essential to focus on strategies that actively promote health and healthy lifestyles and prevent diseases rather than merely treating disease when it occurs. It should be obvious to all that this approach would mean healthier lives for our citizens and a huge reduction in the total cost of health care. (Of course, the cynic will respond that if we live longer, we will incur other costs—diseases later in life that are expensive to treat, more Social Security payments, and other societal expenditures—but most of us would rather live longer and have good health along the way.)

VISION SUMMARY

So what should the vision for tomorrow's health care be? It should be about health, not just diagnosis and treatment of illness. It should focus on protecting, nurturing, and preserving health. It should address our behaviors, our environment, and our social situations so that everyone can have the benefit of a healthy lifetime. We cannot change our genes, but we can understand them, and when disease is predicted, we can plot preventive approaches. We can provide everyone with the available vaccines to prevent infections that maim and kill. We can incentivize physicians and other health-care providers to spend time and energy with each of us and educate us about the best ways to preserve our health or return to a state of good health. We also can incentivize our physicians so that more will become generalists and, with the right opportunities, will want to practice in underserved communities. We can encourage the development of nurse practitioners, physician assistants, pharmacists, social workers, and other health-care providers to augment the role of the generalist physician.

We also need to create incentives for ourselves to live a healthy lifestyle. This point might sound counterintuitive since everyone wants to be healthy, but many of us engage in behaviors that are not conducive to good health, and an incentive system will be critical to help us overcome them. The purpose of the incentives actually is to help us take responsibility for our own health. Good health comes with its own set of responsibilities and requirements.

We recognize that the chronic diseases that now beset our population need a new approach to care, one that addresses long-term, coordinated disease management rather than the episodic interventions that medical care has provided until now. We will insist on team management for complex diseases and arrange our payment systems to ensure it will occur. We can also appreciate that because most complex, chronic diseases are caused by our behaviors and are therefore preventable, our personal behaviors need to change. Regarding our national approach to nutrition and food safety, we need to encourage agriculture to produce quality, nutritious foodstuffs and to empower the USDA and the Food and Drug Administration to make certain foods are free of infection or toxic potential.

In this new vision of health care, we will focus more on the individual thanks to our ability to look at his or her genome, to design individual vaccines, and to plan surgery with the individual's CT scan as a guide. We will set up wellness programs to prevent the diseases for which our genetics put us at risk and use vaccines to prevent not only infections but also chronic diseases like cancer, atherosclerosis, and possibly even Alzheimer's. We will have the ability to repair many failing organs with new and improved approaches from our incredible biomedical research output and with the efforts of engineering and computer scientists to create medical devices, imaging equipment, and operating room (OR) technologies. We will have instantly accessible medical information no matter where we are. We will find ways to dramatically improve patient safety and clinical quality.

And now, understanding what system of care we want for America, let us consider the organizational structure, or the "form" to follow the "function" of our vision. We must come to grips with the uninsured in a manner that not only creates financial coverage but also actually offers real access to providers, especially primary care providers. Then everyone—no matter where they live, what they earn, or what their age—will be ensured complete health care.

With an understanding of the desired system, we can then address the means to pay for it. I would suggest that we require everyone, except the poor, to pay for basic care out of pocket. Everyone would have a high-deductible catastrophic insurance policy that is portable, cannot be cancelled for a preexisting condition, and has no co-pays. We would establish health savings accounts and incentives to encourage us to invest pretax dollars so that we would have the funds to pay for routine care and even predictable yet expensive needs such as drugs, vaccines, colonoscopies, or even routine childbirth. Insurance would pick up the costs whenever they become too burdensome. Also, once the deductible has been reached, insurance would pay not only for hospital and doctor visits but also for e-mail consults, telemedicine, and telediagnosis; for the time needed to coordinate care of chronic illnesses; for preventive care; and for any other aspect of care that is proven of value. We would expect insurance to do so without excess bureaucracy and frustrating delays and denials.

As we modify the current broken medical care system into a true health-care system for all, it is essential that we address the high and rapidly rising costs of care. Only by controlling costs will we have the resources to make the other, necessary changes to ensure better care, better health, and longer, more productive, more satisfying lives. By focusing on preventive care and care coordination along with quality and safety enhancements, we can go a long way toward making care less expensive as well. By correcting the current, perverse insurance arrangements so that the patient has a direct financial contract with the provider, we will have created a strong incentive to improve quality, manage costs, and prevent fraud and abuse.

All of these changes should occur in a setting where the patient comes first and is treated with respect, prompt responses, good communication, and easy access to care and full information. The patient must no longer be marginalized; instead, he or she must become the center of the system. Nothing less will be acceptable in this consumer-driven health-care system.

To achieve this vision will require real leadership, which I define as having three essential steps. First is setting the vision. Next is then persuading all parties involved to commit to realizing the vision. And the final step is getting the key players actually to make it happen. Some of this leadership will need to emanate from our president. It will also require the leadership of those who control much of the funding: the insurance industry, large corporations, unions, and Congress. But we do not have to wait for action from the executive branch and legislators. There is much that individuals and a combination of the leaders in medicine—physicians, hospitals, pharmaceutical firms, and medical device manufacturers—can do immediately. The leaders of Howard County, Maryland, have shown this type of vision where rights and responsibilities coincide. Now we need it nationally.

PART II
MEGATRENDS IN MEDICAL CARE DELIVERY

In this section I will first review the truly amazing advances in science, engineering, and computing that help us understand disease better, offer new approaches to care, and ultimately assist us in preventing illness during our lifetimes. I will then address the delivery of medical care, beginning with important changes in demographics, in the types of illnesses that tend to occur today, and within the health-care system—changes that impact how we receive care and whether that care is of high quality. I will also focus on complex, chronic illnesses and how they fundamentally need new approaches to care delivery.

Some of the coming advances in care might be termed "sustaining," meaning that they are the natural, useful improvements to what we already know or do. Others, however, are truly disruptive or transformational. These developments break new ground, create new paradigms, and overall substantially change or advance what we know, what we do, or how we do it. Many of the advances and changes I will discuss fit this "disruptive" category.

Scientific Advances That Will Affect Health Care—with or without Reform

Misconception: *Health-care reform will have an impact on the advances in medical science.*
George Jones, a middle-aged banker in otherwise good health, had been plagued by digestion difficulties. He had a defect in his diaphragm, the muscle that expands and contracts the lungs and divides the chest from the abdomen, that allowed part of his stomach to push into the chest and to displace his left lung. Surgery was planned, but the surgeon wanted no surprises. I was able to observe how the surgeon planned for the case. A CT scan, using a new multi-slice machine, produced exquisite pictures that rivaled those of an artist. The computer assigned colors to the various organs: blue for the lungs, red for the heart, white for the intestines, and so on. The surgeon looked at the scan and, wanting a better view of the stomach and diaphragm, asked to have the lungs, ribs, intestines, liver, and spleen deleted from the image. At the push of a button, she could see the stomach extending through the diaphragm and could decide whether to operate via an incision in the chest or the abdomen and whether she could do it with the less invasive laparoscopic technique.[1] Next, she transferred the digital CT data into the simulator and practiced the surgery until she felt satisfied. Finally, she uploaded the simulated data into the robot so that it could assist in the actual surgery the next day.

These incredible advances were hardly imagined only a few years ago. They are all related to the research being conducted in medical schools, the medical device industry, and the pharmaceutical and biotechnology industries and are the result of rapid breakthroughs in biologic, engineering, and computer sciences. Health-care reform will neither aid nor abet these types of advances.

The current political debate reflects America's concerns with the status of health-care policy, but another aspect of medicine—its inexorable progress, which will happen no matter what—isn't being discussed. I find this lack of discussion fascinating given that we pride ourselves on our prowess to create innovative approaches. We really need to understand what is happening and what is anticipated in medicine if we want to make rational decisions about what needs to change. Let's begin with the amazing scientific advances in medicine that are and will be here soon regardless of the federal changes as part of health-care reform.

Several medical megatrends will profoundly affect medical care delivery. Some will stem from the explosion of basic understandings of cellular and molecular biology while others are related to developments in engineering and computer science. Altogether they will create five huge shifts in medicine:

1.   Custom-tailored medicine
2.   Much greater emphasis on prevention
3.   Improved ability to repair, restore function to, or replace organs, tissues, or cells
4.   Fully digitized medical records available instantly anytime, anyplace
5.   Enhanced level of safety and quality of care

A common misconception is that reform will impact such medical advances. In actuality, the reforms from Washington will not affect them much (except for the electronic medical record), yet these changes will profoundly impact the care we receive in the near future. They are truly disruptive in that medicine will be forever different as a result.

What is driving these disruptive megatrends?[2] First, advances in biomedical research are resulting in medical improvements. The science of genomics, a word few knew and fewer still understood early in the twenty-first century, has opened a new era in medicine. Understanding deoxyribonucleic acid (DNA), the code of life, will allow us to predict diseases that will occur in later years but could be prevented if dealt with now; to create drugs targeted at a specific molecular focus; to prescribe a drug for an individual that will definitively work with few if any side effects; and to assay whether a disease such as a cancer will recur after a course of therapy. Fundamentally, genomics represents a revolution in medical discovery and opportunities for care. In addition, our knowledge of stem cells will continue to advance. Already stem cells are used in treating and occasionally curing some forms of leukemia, and preliminary studies are focusing on stem cells administered after a heart attack in hopes of restoring cardiac muscles and small blood vessels. Eventually, stem cells will be available on demand for the individual whose loss of islet cells in the pancreas has created type 1 diabetes mellitus. With good luck and much discovery work, stem cells may be able to cure Parkinson's disease and possibly even spinal cord injury. The opportunities are legion, but I caution you to recognize that our knowledge base today is limited. Stem cells remain a promise for the future, not a panacea for tomorrow. Further, there are, of course, ethical issues involved in working specifically with embryonic stem cells, and the politicization of these issues may well prevent this future resource from coming to fruition.

New vaccines, courtesy of advances in immunology, prevent such infections as herpes zoster (shingles) in later years and rotavirus-induced severe diarrhea in infants and toddlers. We can expect more new vaccines for infection prevention, and many will be administered by patch, by mouth, or by nasal spray rather than by shots. Two new vaccines prevent cancer—the hepatitis vaccine, which prevents hepatoma, a common liver cancer in many parts of the world; and the new vaccine to prevent human papillomavirus (HPV) infection, which causes cervical cancer in women. The latter vaccine may prove useful in preventing anal cancer (the type of cancer Farrah Fawcett developed) and some cancers of the mouth and throat. I predict the development of vaccines to prevent some leukemias and lymphomas and stomach cancer within ten to fifteen years. Eventually, vaccines will also help treat cancer. A prostate cancer treatment vaccine was approved in 2010 by the FDA, and others are being evaluated for colon cancer, breast cancer, and, of course, HIV-AIDS. I am especially excited that we can look for vaccines over the next decade or two to help treat many chronic diseases, such as multiple sclerosis and type 1 diabetes, and to help prevent Alzheimer's, atherosclerosis (which leads to heart attacks and strokes), and possibly even drug addiction. One day a "designer" vaccine may even be tailor made to treat your specific cancer, as is the case with the new prostate vaccine called Provenge.

Today patients in need of transplants receive organs (kidney, lung, liver, heart, intestine, and pancreas) from donors who have died, usually in auto accidents, but there are never enough organs to treat the many patients who need them. Some will receive a kidney or a part of a liver from a living donor; this is obviously not possible with all organ transplants, such as hearts. Most people in need of a heart transplant die before an organ becomes available. But in the not-too-distant future, surgeons will use xenotransplantation, which involves taking an organ from an animal rather than a human, so that a patient will get it immediately and not need to wait and "hope" for someone else to die. The animal, most likely a pig, will be bred and raised so that its organs will not excite our bodies to try to eradicate, or "reject," it. As a result, expensive and potentially toxic antirejection drugs will no longer be needed.

In the future, we may come to think of the new hospital blood bank as the "farm" where animals grown for their organs and stem cells are produced in mass numbers for patients in need.

Just as basic medical science is advancing toward custom-tailored treatments and preventive efforts, engineering and computer science are also making medical procedures safer. In fact, while we often think of most medical progress as stemming from the NIH research labs, the pharmaceutical or biotech industries, or our medical schools over the past fifty years, we must also recognize the incredible advances that have come from engineering and computer science. Imaging has progressed dramatically, for one; today's CT scanners produce exquisite pictures of our anatomy. Coronary arteries can be visualized on their insides—a view once seen only with the invasive angiography technique—and detect obstructions, helping emergency room doctors diagnose the cause of chest pain. Many individuals who come to the ER with chest pain have negative or equivocal electrocardiograms, and the newer CT scanner answers whether they have coronary artery disease within a few minutes. In addition, it can reveal other life-threatening conditions that cause chest pain such as an aortic aneurysm, pneumonia, or even gallstones. This major advance markedly improves rapid diagnosis.

Digitally recorded images can be manipulated and visualized in three dimensions, and organs can be rendered in different colors to get a clearer view. As described in the vignette at the beginning of this chapter, every good surgeon will tell you that he or she does not want any surprises during surgery, but they happen frequently. Think of the advantages to the surgeon who will now know exactly what anatomy to expect before beginning an operation.

Increasingly, molecular changes in our cells will be detected and reported as an image. For example, we will be able to differentiate whether a cancer has spread or whether it has regressed after chemotherapy using positron emission tomography (PET) scans or other newer approaches. Functions in the brain can be visualized while they are happening using functional magnetic resonance imaging (fMRI) or PET scans. We now can "see" thoughts in progress.

Engineering and computer science advances have led to the creation of medical devices that are smaller and more powerful with long battery life. Former vice president Dick Cheney's implanted heart defibrillator and his left ventricular assist device are examples. So, too, are similarly implanted devices that go into the vagus nerve, which travels down the neck from the brain, and that send tiny electrical impulses upstream to help reduce epileptic attacks or improve serious depression. Diabetics can now wear on their belts pumps the size of a cigarette box that deliver insulin at the right rate, and the closed-loop models in development will be able to monitor blood sugar continuously and tell the pump how much insulin to inject. No more finger sticks!

Among the other examples of rapid advances, in the field of nanomedicine, researchers are developing submicroscopic devices. For example, a molecularly sized "device" will be able to search out and attach itself to hidden cancer cells, emit a signal to allow the detection and imaging of the cells' location, and carry a substance (radiation or chemical) to kill them. It will be a three-in-one tool to knock out the hidden cancer cells. Meanwhile, huge machines, such as radiation therapy electron accelerators, will be increasingly able to target a tumor while sparing the adjoining normal tissues, resulting in a more effective and much safer treatment. Among many other new devices is a big advance for the amputee, an artificial hand. Driven by a computer chip and multiple tiny motors at each knuckle, its fingers are capable of grasping a soda can, pressing the buttons of a touch pad phone or automated teller machine (ATM), and grasping an object with the thumb and forefinger. In the area of infection diagnosis, it will be possible to take a microscopic sample and determine the germ (bacteria, virus, fungus, and so on) causing the infection along with its susceptibility to various antimicrobials all in an hour or two.

The operating room is now a technological marvel and will become even more so. But first consider that less work needs to be done in the OR. Ulcers, for instance, once the main occupation of the general surgeon, are now permanently cured with a combination of drugs that eradicates the *Helicobacter pylori* (*H. pylori*) bacteria that causes them. More surgeries will be done in less invasive manners, such as those performed in the radiology suite, where doctors insert tiny catheters via a patient's vein or artery in the groin, advance them to a site of disease, and correct it without typical surgery. For example, for years the standard approach to treating aortic aneurysms involved a major operation requiring many postoperative days in the ICU, a week in the hospital, and then a month of recuperation. Now it takes an hour or so to place the graft via catheter, and the patient goes home the next day with little or no recuperation time and few of the risks associated with major surgery. A similar example is used to ablate a brain aneurysm; the doctor inserts platinum coils in the aneurysm to clog it off, stopping it from bleeding into the brain and preventing a major stroke. The formerly tried-and-true approach was to open the skull (a craniotomy), find the vessel with its aneurysm deep in the brain, and then put a silver clip across it. This operation was obviously a major procedure with many risks that required a significant hospital stay. But the catheter approach is relatively quick, requires no open surgery, and boasts a rapid recovery time.

Soon some surgery, such as gall bladder removal, may be done through natural orifices. Doctors using an endoscopic surgical device with a controlled "robotic" arm at the end will insert it into the patient's mouth and down into the stomach. It then goes through the stomach wall, finds the gall bladder, and removes it. This technique is used also to remove the appendix by inserting the endoscopic instruments via the vagina or possibly the rectum, leaving no scars and allowing faster healing.

Just as an airline pilot practices in a flight simulator before ever sitting in the cockpit, so, too, will surgical trainees demonstrate their competency before ever operating on a person. Master surgeons will use an individual patient's own CT scan inserted into the simulator and practice a specific surgical approach. Robots will assist the surgeon based on the information uploaded from the simulated practice; the robot never gets tired, doesn't have a hand tremor, does not feel sore from leaning over the operating room table, and can be programmed for "no fly zones," or specific areas not to venture into even if the surgeon, who is always in control of the robot, accidentally directs it do so. So all of these and more will mean better quality and great safety.

And, at last, the time will come in five to fifteen years when all medical information, from your doctor's office notes to images for the surgery, will be digitized and available in your medical record. Wherever you are, your medical information will be available instantly via the Internet, a chip on a card in your wallet, or on a flash memory device such as those used in cell phones and digital cameras and now worn by some of American soldiers as a dog tag.

We will see complementary medicine practices, such as acupuncture, meditation, massage, and some herbal remedies, become part of the regimen of care as they are taught more and more in medical school and are subjected to the same types of scientific analyses as other medical techniques. We already know that acupuncture, for example, can help relieve lower back pain or the pain of osteoarthritis of the knee. Meditation, as part of a total program, can assist in relieving stress and with it the risk of coronary artery damage.

Medical care as outlined in this chapter is changing rapidly. It will continue to do so because of the convergence of laboratory discoveries, engineering skills and computational power, entrepreneurial focus, and the ability to patent intellectual property. Reviewing the five disruptive megatrends, genomics will enable care to become custom tailored by helping your doctor choose the right medicine for you and alerting you to the risk of disease in the future. Stem cells will be prepared to combat your particular personal illness, and an animal will be raised with an organ that will correct your specific problem. You might get a designer vaccine for your type of cancer, and your surgeon will know exactly what to expect during surgery after checking your radiographic images.

Your genomic information, vaccines to prevent chronic illnesses, and drugs chosen to be effective while avoiding side effects will boost your efforts at disease prevention. Your cells, tissues, and organs will be repaired, restored to normal function, or replaced with new surgical techniques, new pharmaceuticals, gene therapy, transplantation, or nano-medical devices.

You will always have your medical record available, when traveling or when referred to a specialist. The care you receive will be safer because providers will have been trained and then certified on a simulator; a robot will assist the surgeon and genomics will tell the physician what medication to use or avoid for you.

These five megatrends are inevitable, albeit the time frame for each will certainly vary. Unfortunately, the delivery of health care has not kept pace with the new advances in medical science and technology. Often the provider is either unaware of the new approaches, has not learned how to use them, or is not cognizant of their benefits. As well, health policy lags behind our medical knowledge and abilities. As the reforms from Washington take place, they will likely not affect the development of our new knowledge to prevent, slow, or cure disease.

— 5 —

Surprising Drivers of Change in Health-Care Delivery

Misconception: *Health-care reform will improve the delivery of care and offer us better care opportunities.*

Albert Meriwether (here and elsewhere the names of individuals and certain possible identifying characteristics have been changed to preserve anonymity) had never been to doctors much, but he did have good health insurance through his unionized position at the shipyards in Baltimore. Now retired for a few years, he was a widower and lived alone. He had few friends and no social networks although his daughter visited occasionally on weekends. Mostly he sat on the living-room couch, watched TV, drank beer, smoked cigarettes, and ate popcorn and potato chips. His weight rose dramatically in retirement, reaching 438 pounds. His daughter called one Sunday and reported that her father had suffered a heart attack, that he had been taken to a nearby community hospital, and that the cardiologist wanted him to have open-heart surgery as soon as possible. He preferred a surgeon at the University of Maryland Medical Center, but, unfortunately, he reported, no beds were available that weekend so the surgery would have to wait. Was there anything I could do to speed his transfer?

I made a call to the senior vice president of patient care services, and Mr. Meriwether was brought over later that afternoon and had his surgery first thing Monday morning. (I wondered but never asked if someone else had been denied a berth because of my call or if the "found" bed had been vacant all along.) At the end of the day on Monday, I went to visit him. On the way I bumped into the surgeon who told me, with a devious grin on his face, that everything had gone well but it was good that he "had long arms." He explained that because Mr. Meriwether was exceedingly obese, "it was a long way in to get to his heart." As it turned out, he did fine and was ready for discharge shortly. When I asked where he would go, we learned that his insurance did not cover any form of cardiac rehabilitation so he would be going home—home to the couch, the beer, and the potato chips.

What a waste, I thought. Here he had recently received a $60,000 "plumbing job," but no one would spend a few more dollars to ensure that he would not be back again shortly and in need of more expensive repairs. Our system of care is so focused on disease treatment that it neglects promoting wellness and prevention and obtaining the most value from the treatments we give. Instead, it focuses on the disease once it has caused havoc, and then only acutely, rather than on preventing it or dealing with it in a better way, usually with relatively inexpensive approaches.

Mr. Meriwether's story represents many of the problems of our system today and why I call it a medical care rather than a health-care system. Mr. Meriwether needed preventive care years before his heart attack and postoperative care coordination with cardiac rehabilitation after his discharge. Meanwhile, the system spent huge amounts of money on his acute, immediate medical care but was not equipped to work on and maintain his health.

The delivery of medical care, as with the scientific advances discussed in chapter 4, is undergoing rapid changes. Some are for the better, some not. Today's common misconception is that health-care reform will improve how we receive care. In actuality, reform will probably have little impact; but medical care delivery is going to change rather dramatically because key shifts in society and demographics along with a marked difference in the most common types of serious illnesses that we will develop will drive delivery modifications. To appreciate these developments, it is worthwhile to consider what our health-care system looks like now and what is happening that will alter it substantially in the coming years. These changes are coming and are inevitable. They will occur at different rates, but they will happen. Similar to the medical changes we will see from scientific advances, these changes in health-care delivery too will be disruptive megatrends.

SOME OVERARCHING PERSPECTIVES ABOUT OUR HEALTH-CARE SYSTEM

Let's consider the dominant perspectives of our health-care system today and then look at some of the drivers of change in the system. Chapter 6 will detail the results of that change, or what we can expect as major trends in the future.

Again, we have to recognize that America truly has a "sick care system" rather than a health-care system, meaning that insurance, doctors, and hospitals focus on disease and injury. Further, the system places little emphasis on prevention, wellness, and health maintenance today, and frankly doctors and hospitals have no incentives to do so. American medical care is expensive, yet it does not achieve what we might call "peer" standards, as I noted regarding infant mortality and life expectancy (see chapter 2). The medical industry is strongly protective of its financial well-being and will allow change only after great difficulty and pressure. Further, I believe that professionalism among medical providers to some degree is eroding. Too many are in the health-care professions for the money rather than for the joy of helping others.[1]

We have an aging population, and older people simply will experience more illness in the future as their "old parts wear out." More and more, disease today is chronic, complex, and lifelong rather than being acute and short lived. We lead unhealthy lifestyles, which in turn will beget substantially more chronic, lifelong illnesses in the coming years.

Although we undertake enormous efforts in basic medical science ($30 billion per year with the National Institutes of Health), these efforts mostly address illness, not health matters. Our public health system, where we spend relatively little, is in disrepair. And while we as individuals are changing our perceptions of and expectations for medical care—we expect to be treated as consumers of services who can go elsewhere if unsatisfied—the delivery system's focus is on the provider. Although our politicians have passed health-care reform, it does not address health issues; rather, it covers medical care financing. Finally, we need to recognize that change tends to be incremental in American medicine. Despite our desires, we should not anticipate radical change occurring rapidly without a precipitating crisis or major shift in political willpower.

DRIVERS OF CHANGE IN MEDICAL CARE DELIVERY

Some of the possible future drivers of change in the delivery of medical care are reflected in the following list. While there will always be many advances in medicine—new drugs and new technologies—we will also see new approaches to care. Sometimes an advance is revolutionary or disruptive. We are in a period now with many truly disruptive changes occurring.

Scientific Advances

In chapter 4, I reviewed some scientific advances that will drive the disruptive megatrends in the delivery of medical care. They include genomics, stem cells, xenotransplantation, miniaturized devices and nanomedicine, interventional radiology, among others.

Growth in Demand for Medical Services

Although medicine has for many, many years focused on episodes of acute care requirements, such as trauma, acute appendicitis, pneumonia, or the need to remove a gall bladder, today more and more of medicine focuses on chronic diseases. Heart failure, diabetes, cancer, multiple sclerosis, arthritis, lupus, and other diseases are with us for many years, often for life, and require different types of medical services. They drive greater numbers of patients to seek more care. I cannot overemphasize the importance of this change in disease patterns as it will have a major impact on how medicine is delivered, what medical care is delivered, and how that care will be financed. I also cannot stress enough that much of this rise of complex, chronic illness directly results from our personal behaviors.

Additionally, as more people survive longer, they will face more medical problems, many of which will require medical interventions within intensive care settings. The intensive care units within hospitals then will have to expand. That said, many other interventions now can be performed in less intense settings. Interventional radiologists, for example, are doing many procedures that previously had to be done in the operating room. Other surgical procedures—such as cataract, knee repair, or hernia surgery—are now carried out in ambulatory settings. Operations with long incisions that once required a lengthy hospital stay afterward, such as the removal of a gall bladder, can now be done with laparoscopic surgery, and the patient goes home the same or the next day. These incredible advances will help drive how medical care is delivered in the future. But despite these newfound abilities to do more outside the hospital walls or the OR, more and more individuals will need the high technology of the ICU because the nature of their illnesses will require these specialized, intense settings. Concurrently they will need the "high touch" of dedicated nurses and physicians to assure the best care; technology alone is not sufficient for superior care.

Financial Issues

Multiple financial issues also will drive future changes in how medical care is delivered. First among them are the rapidly rising costs of medical care. In the United States we now spend more than 17 percent of our GDP on medical care, and medical

care inflation has increased around 10 percent per year, or well above general inflation. Yet, despite these expenditures, 47 million fellow Americans are uninsured.
This statistic is remarkable given the increased number of people insured by government programs, particularly children, since the year 2000. Of course, as a result of
reform legislation, this number of uninsured will begin to change as many of these
individuals will become eligible for Medicaid and others will no longer be rejected
for insurance because of preexisting conditions or exceeding lifetime limits.

Despite all the funds spent on medical care, though, those who do have what
is considered good insurance coverage for medical care usually lack coverage or have
inadequate coverage for preventive care, rehabilitation, sub-acute care, and home
health-care programs. This circumstance is also curious given that these programs
actually bring down the total cost of health care. The same issue applies to "e" medicine. Most insurance plans do not reimburse providers for using e-mail, telemedicine, telediagnosis, and related approaches, yet they could reduce the need for office
visits, prevent hospitalizations, and decrease costs overall while improving patients'
outcomes and quality of life. Further, insurers are carefully restricting access—access
to drugs, access to hospitals, access to specialists. They take these steps to try to reduce rapidly rising health-care costs, but in the end insurers find that patients, hospitals, and doctors all rebel, at least to the extent possible. The result is that Americans
spend an enormous amount for medical care, yet we receive neither the preventive
care and wellness care to maintain our health nor the benefits of our physicians' attention for prevention and care coordination that could actually help us reduce the
costs of care.

RISING COSTS OF CONSTRUCTION AND TECHNOLOGY

With more of us surviving longer and with more complex, chronic diseases developing, we will need additional hospitals and beds. But the costs of construction
and technology are rising rapidly and faster than general inflation is. The costs are
incredibly expensive for imaging machines such as CT scanners and MRI scanners,
for medical devices such as pacemakers and cardiac stents, and for pharmaceuticals
such as those used for cancer care and multiple sclerosis.

Consumerism

Meanwhile, patient expectations will increase exponentially. In this new consumerism, patients will expect service, safety, quality, and respect, or they will go to a differ-

ent doctor or a different hospital. Right now, consumers are indicating they are less than satisfied with the system of care.

When patients are surveyed regarding their perception of satisfaction with their hospital care, it correlates fairly well with the quality of care at that hospital.[2] Few hospitals receive high marks from 90 percent or more of their discharged patients. The most frequent areas of patient concern or complaint are nursing care, communication about medications, pain control, and the provision of clear discharge instructions. The bottom line is that patients feel there is plenty of room for improvement.

The American health-care system also earns poor marks when compared with those of the other thirty-three countries of the Organization for Economic Cooperation and Development (OECD).[3] In surveys, individuals with chronic illness report higher out-of-pocket expenses that often adversely affect their care, many problems with care coordination (such as records or test results not being available at a scheduled appointment), and more medical errors. Apparently among those patients with chronic diseases, America stands out compared to other OECD countries for having the most negative experiences.

When assessing their expectations, according to patients, convenience will matter, including short travel distances. Responsiveness of the staff, brief waiting periods, and easy access will be critical. Providers' communication and responsiveness will also be essential, for patients will expect their physicians to respond to e-mails and text messages and to do so in a reasonably short time. Future patients will expect pleasant yet informed discussions, not pro forma pronouncements or vague explanations of diseases or treatments. Indeed, absent satisfaction on these counts, patients will look to alternatives as the patient with breast cancer did in chapter 1. This assertiveness is a real change. In the past, patients tolerated long waits to get an appointment, put up with short visits despite unresolved issues, accepted their providers' pronouncements without query, and were loath to change providers. So this new consumerism will be a major driver of change into the future. Departing from the way medicine was done in the past is disruptive. No longer will the patient be willing to be patient.

There are certain principles of patient and family-centered care. First, treat the individual with respect and dignity. Second, share unbiased information in a useful format. Third, invite the patient and his or her family to participate in the decision making based on the information available. And finally, have good collaboration among the patient, the family, and the providers. While not an unreasonable set of goals, they are different from the way medicine has been practiced to a large degree in the past. Basically patients want the following: respect for their preferences and values, coordination of care, communication, physical comfort, emotional support as needed, family and friends' involvement, continuity, and easy access to their care and care providers.[4]

At the same time hospital boards of trustees will need to change their approach substantially. Over the years, trustees of community hospitals have been the paragons of the community, chosen largely because of their business successes, their interest in civic activities, and perhaps their ability to make sizable donations. But in the future, trustees will need to address issues that they have not fully addressed in the past. Yes, they will still have to handle the financial status of the hospital, but now they also will focus extensively on consumerism, quality, and safety. Previously, most board members have been uncomfortable with these issues. A trustee would say, "How can I address quality and safety when I don't have a medical background?" But government regulators and patients will demand that trustees focus with real metrics and real attention to quality and safety. As consumerism begins to take hold in medicine, look for hospital trustees to be chosen not only on the criteria of the past but also because of their interest and willingness to examine programs for quality and safety, to be attentive to consumerism, to maintain the nonprofit status of their institutions, and yet still be attentive to the financial necessities of the institution.

Professional Issues

Clearly there is and will be a significant shortage of physicians. As the population increases and ages, our medical schools are not producing enough physicians to provide the necessary care. But the situation is more complex. About as many women as men are now graduating from medical school, and many of these women will want to take time out for raising a family. This creates another form of short-term shortage, whether they work part time or not at all for some years. Medical school is very expensive. Public medical schools average $44,000 per year in tuition, fees, and living expenses; private schools average $62,000 per year. Most students begin their practice with a substantial debt of $100,000 or more. Indeed, the median debt load for graduates of public medical schools is $145,000 and of private medical schools is $180,000, with about a quarter of graduates accumulating a debt load of more than $200,000.[5]

About 70 percent of American physicians are specialists and 30 percent are generalists. In most other countries this ratio is reversed. This shift is largely owing to our insurance reimbursement mechanisms, which encourage specialization by paying the specialist more. A general internist in private practice for about ten years earns about $150,000 per year whereas a general surgeon may bring home double that amount. So pay differences and a high debt lead new graduates to choose a specialization. In addition, physicians' lifestyle expectations are changing. For example, medical staff traditionally accepted emergency room "on call status" on a rotating basis. Young physicians starting out used the experience as a way to build up their practices. But now physicians won't do that kind of work unless the hospital will actually pay them to be on call because too many patients either do not have insurance or are unable to pay out of pocket. While the physicians do not mind taking the occasional patient who cannot pay, nowadays so many uninsured people use the ER for their primary care that the system is "out of balance."

More and more physicians now are forgoing private practice to be employed or to enter a contractual arrangement. In part, this choice allows them to have a steadier income stream, but it also addresses a quality of life issue by allotting more personal and family time. Being employed means the physician does not have to worry about the overhead of an office or the costs of malpractice insurance, although they soon learn from the practice manager that they still must see a certain number of patients per day in order to maintain their income. In other words, they shortly learn that no matter what form of practice they have, there are obligations and responsibilities to assure their income. These changes in lifestyle expectations are also causing many physicians to leave their solo or group practices and to begin working for hospitals, HMOs, or large groups. Even though a general surgeon may earn more than an internist does, the surgeon also finds that making that income requires long hours and many nights in the operating room. Many instead are saying, "No, thanks." As with primary care physicians, this trend is impacting rural and urban poor areas the most.

Not everyone believes a serious physician shortage is pending. Some argue that if medical care were better coordinated and ancillary caregivers better utilized, then the country would have plenty of physicians. I doubt this assumption is correct, but it is worth discussion. Certainly, better coordination is seriously needed (see chapters 6 and 9), and we could make wider use of nurse practitioners, physician assistants, social workers, and others (chapter 9). Meanwhile, whether primary care or specialist, physicians are all frustrated with low reimbursements from insurers, with major hassles and barriers erected by insurers, and with the need for a larger office staff simply to keep up with the insurers' bureaucracy.

A significant shortage of nurses, pharmacists, and many other health-care providers already exists. The average age of nurses in a hospital has been steadily increasing because not enough new nurses are coming into the workforce, despite the rise in salaries. The number of nurses, mostly employed by hospitals, rose from 2 million to about 2.35 million between 2001 and 2007. But interestingly, much of this increase came from older registered nurses (RNs) entering the workforce, presumably from other occupations, and from a major influx of foreign-born nurses.[6] Work content and work expectations have been changing as well, and many nurses feel that they spend too much time dealing with required documentation and other mandates and all too little time at the actual patient's bedside. Nurses, like physicians, want their family time and are less willing to accept rotating shifts where they have to take their share of evening or night work. A nurse I know who used to work at a nearby community hospital became so fed up with all of the paperwork and other "busy work" that she quit and joined a home cleaning service. She observed, "I make less money as a maid but I don't go home frustrated every night that I could not give my patients the care they deserved and that I knew I could give if I just had the time." Others are remaining in the medical care field but are gravitating to non-patient care roles such as case managers or taking jobs in ambulatory care settings where the pressures are less demanding. To be complete, there is just now a temporary hiatus in the nurse shortage with more nurses graduating and fewer retiring as a result of the current economic stagnation. But the shortage will shortly reappear.

A trend once again toward a larger nurse to patient ratio stems in part from the recognition that nurses are key to improved patient safety and medical care quality. The hospital workplace is beginning to gravitate toward a more satisfying venue for the nurse. But despite the slight increase in graduates entering the workforce, the rate of the older nurses' retirements will largely offset this advance, leaving a net shortage while hospitals project the need for more nurses in the coming years. This scenario suggests a need for nursing programs to produce greater numbers of RNs.

As for pharmacists, the shortages are also growing. Most pharmacy schools have changed the curriculum, and instead of offering a master's degree they now offer the PharmD degree. Its requirement adds a year to the curriculum and produces a better-educated and better-trained graduate. These pharmacists are better positioned to add to the patient's understanding of the drugs prescribed and to watch for drug-drug interactions that might be a safety issue. This aspect is particularly important for patients with complex, chronic diseases who may well be taking ten or more medicines. Finally, these new PharmD graduates have different work expectations than those of their predecessors and anticipate having more interaction and time with patients. Hospitals and pharmacies will need to address those new notions.

Patient Responsibility

One of the biggest drivers of change in future health-care delivery will be increased patient responsibility. As employers face rapidly rising health-care costs, they expect their employees to pay an increasing percentage of the insurance. The insurers have added deductibles and co-pays so that the individual is paying for a greater share of the cost of care. Many companies now offer medical savings accounts, and those who buy their insurance individually with a high deductible can enroll in health savings accounts. Both types of accounts allow the individual to use pretax dollars to pay for the deductibles and co-pays, but it all means the patient takes greater responsibility both for his or her own care and for paying for it.

SUMMARY

We can expect a substantially increased demand for medical services accompanied by rising costs for medical care. Already we have seen a big rise in the cost of constructing new facilities and for technology purchases. Our insurance system for reimbursing medical care will be another driver of change, as will the national issue of providing coverage for the underinsured and uninsured. The interaction of medicine with computer science and engineering will rapidly advance and impact care in ways far greater than most of us appreciate today.

Americans are waking up and insisting that medical providers should show them respect, even if they do not pay the providers directly. In the end, through lost wages and taxes, however, they are the ones paying the bills from the physician, nurse, other providers, and the hospital. In meeting consumers' demands, medicine will need to demonstrate quality and safety; however, at the same time, physicians, nurses, pharmacists, and other health-care professionals will be in short supply. We will also witness some substantial changes in what physicians, nurses, and others expect from their careers in health care.

Another major change driving the delivery of health care is that patients will take greater and greater responsibility for their own care and paying for it. We will also see greater responsibility placed on hospital trustees, and we will see the government increase the amount of regulation and mandates in the coming years.

6

The Tsunami Is Coming

Misconception: *The remarkable advances from the basic biological, engineering, and computer sciences are rapidly made available to the medical care delivery system and to the patients who can most benefit from them.*

I served on a committee to evaluate a new academic hospital under construction. After reviewing the architectural blueprints, the technology programs, and other materials, I asked about the plans for simulation laboratories, because from what I saw, the architects had not allocated any space for them. The CEO said that they were not in the current plans since the affiliated medical school had a facility that could be used, although it was some miles away. He did not seem to feel having a simulation lab was critical for the new facility. My understanding of the value of simulation suggested that these facilities should be readily accessible and immediately adjacent to the procedural areas, such as the operating rooms, the cardiac catheterization laboratory, and the gastrointestinal endoscopy area. Simulation has come late to medicine, but it is gaining traction for teaching techniques from the simple, such as blood drawing, to the most complex, such as laparoscopic surgery. Simulation allows the trainee to practice repeatedly until he or she is competent rather than "learning on the patient." Locating the training area near the actual procedural area such as the OR is important because trainees can easily access the equipment whenever they have time available. Adjacency also means that expert physicians can gain new technologic prowess and even practice special procedures before their actual cases. Being some distance away, though, ensures that the lab will not be used.

That evening, in January 2009, I mentioned to my wife that I needed to figure out a strong argument for having the labs in the hospital. She gave me the answer.

At our meeting the next day, I asked if anyone believed that the captain of the US Airways flight that had landed in the Hudson River the day before had ever previously landed a plane with both engines out. From the looks on their faces, two of the architects in the room understood where I was going although at least two of the physicians did not. I then pointed out that the pilot in fact had practiced in a cockpit simulator multiple times many different emergency scenarios, including the loss of all power. At three thousand feet with sudden power loss, he did not have time to pull out his manual; he needed to respond immediately based on practical, not book, training. Simulation ensured he knew what to do. Point made.

Unfortunately, although simulation technologies are available now, many hospitals have not purchased them, not wanting to take on "an added cost." Further, many physicians fall back on tradition, saying, "That's not the way we train people here."

The practice of medicine evolves slowly, but sometimes new forces or new technologies or new knowledge lead to disruptive and, indeed, revolutionary change. Such is the case with robotics, genomics, and, quite probably, nanomedicine. Simulation will be very disruptive, changing our centuries-old approach to teaching medicine by practicing first on a patient to now demonstrating competency first on the simulator.

MEDICAL CARE DELIVERY MEGATRENDS

PATIENTS

> older, sicker, greater numbers

HOSPITALS

> more beds, more ICUs, more ORs
>
> use of hospitalists
>
> growth of systems
>
> more use of rehabilitation, sub-acute care, hospice, and home health care

PROFESSIONAL ISSUES

> more use of nonphysician professionals
>
> expectations for better lifestyle
>
> malpractice
>
> restructuring staff

CONSUMERISM

> patient no longer patient

URGENT AND EMERGENT ILLNESSES

COMPLEX, CHRONIC ILLNESSES
>discipline versus disease approach to care
>multidisciplinary teams

REGIONAL ECHELONS OF CARE

DIGITIZED MEDICAL INFORMATION

USE OF TECHNOLOGY
>social media
>avatars

SAFETY AND QUALITY
>simulation
>robotics
>nanotechnology
>evidence-based care
>trustees

ACADEMIC MEDICAL CENTERS
>strengths and weaknesses
>opportunities versus disadvantages

PATIENTS

In coming years, as noted previously, hospitalized patients will be older, sicker, and greater in number. They will be older because more of us are living longer, and with the Baby Boomers moving into retirement years, that trend will be accelerated. Patients will be sicker in part because the increased numbers of older individuals will have a greater number of illnesses, mostly chronic. Although our ability to care for people outside the hospital setting is rapidly advancing, the greater numbers that will still need hospitalization also will be sicker than before. And it is often the case that a person with one chronic illness has another one or two, often related to each other. For example, a patient who has had a heart attack may also be at risk for a stroke or have a reduced blood supply to the legs—all of which are related to atherosclerosis manifested in many parts of the body. Similarly a patient with diabetes may have heart disease, kidney disease, or lower leg arterial disease. These co-morbidities result in a sicker patient. These patients with complex chronic illnesses are the ones who will not only put greater demands on the medical care delivery system but will also need and thereby influence scientific as well as the delivery system advances.

HOSPITALS: BEDS AND CARE

Contradicting the long-held belief that we need fewer hospitals and fewer beds, more hospital units, with most being ICUs, and sophisticated ORs will be constructed to accommodate the increasing numbers of patients. Further, in this setting, there will be multiple approaches to interdigitate the specialists and their functions with new technologies. For example, the electronic intensive care unit (eICU) will become commonplace. A specialist will be present physically some of the time and present virtually all of the time through various forms of distance medicine and telemedicine. This innovation will improve the care of patients, decrease costs, and reduce staffing needs. In particular, these highly trained physicians will be in short supply to begin with, so using their time and expertise via telemedicine techniques will be beneficial to more patients, the hospital, and the wallet.

In all likelihood there will be a big change in what individual hospitals do to consolidate advanced care into a limited number of tertiary care centers. It is simply not practical for smaller hospitals to have all of the costly technologies that are becoming available. Care will increasingly utilize these new technologies, such as the new imaging modalities that cost more than $1 million per piece of equipment. Yet this evolution will be resisted since no hospital or physician wants to be required to "give up" the care of many of their patients.

The use of "hospitalists," another trend in medical care delivery, will continue to expand. A relatively new phenomenon, a hospitalist is a physician who chooses only to take care of patients who are hospitalized. On the one hand, the hospitalist model offers many advantages. The physician hospitalist knows and understands the hospital well and can maneuver within the system in a more effective and efficient manner. Hospitalists can focus on those issues in medicine that arise during the hospital stay and as a result become more proficient. Concurrently, the primary care physician is not called away from his or her office practice during the middle of a busy session and can stay fully focused on outpatient medicine. On the other hand, there are disadvantages with the hospitalist model. Most important, the hospitalist does not know the patient from long experience of annual and routine visits and so does not know the unique aspects of the patient's family life, home setting, work, psychosocial factors, and the like. Second, and somewhat related, is a distinct opportunity for losing data during the handoff process from the primary care physician to the hospitalist at the time of admission and again when the patient is discharged back to the PCP. A good electronic medical record system that integrates both inpatient and outpatient information would mitigate some aspects of this issue although certainly not all of them. A third and related disadvantage is the hospitalist might give expert care to the acute problem that led to the patient's admission, but he or she might not do as well with the long-standing care of the patient's many chronic conditions, a care plan that the PCP has shaped by trial and experience over time.

HOSPITAL SYSTEMS

With more hospitalized patients, with more hospitals and hospital beds being constructed, and with new approaches to patient care, particularly those requiring more intensive care, hospital systems will continue to develop. By "systems" I mean a group of multiple hospitals with the individual hospitals being owned by a parent (not-for-profit or for-profit) corporation or being held together through various partnership arrangements. These systems will continue to grow, largely to access the capital markets. The recent credit market turmoil may actually hasten these consolidations. Hospitals need dollars for construction, and it is harder for a smaller, stand-alone hospital to achieve that access. Similarly it is hard for the smaller, stand-alone hospital to get capital for major technology acquisitions, such as the new CT scanners, the EMR, and the advanced OR technologies. It is not unreasonable to assume that the day of the independent community hospital is rapidly coming to an end.

Geographically oriented hospital systems may also come together to develop logical echelons of care. In this arrangement, the smaller hospitals agree to transfer critically ill individuals immediately to the larger, more comprehensive hospital for definitive care with the understanding that the total system will balance out the funding needs of all. In some cases, and absent a hospital system, the state or another political entity will create a cooperative system to care for certain types of patients, especially those facing acute situations that need emergency medical care such as severe trauma, strokes, and heart attacks.

These geographic systems may vertically integrate by also having a full continuum of services connected to them in some way so they can move patients promptly to the right level of care as their treatment progresses. This arrangement might take the form of an in-system rehabilitation hospital, home health-care agency, and hospice care. A rehabilitation hospital can service a large region and accept discharges from many general hospitals. Rehabilitation depends on using large physical therapy treatment areas where patients mingle and work on issues side by side. This treatment is best done in a separate hospital as opposed to a wing of a general hospital. Meanwhile, sub-acute care works well and creatively within the four walls of the general hospital. The sub-acute unit allows for the early discharge of a patient from the usual inpatient unit to a setting that is less intense and more focused on the patient's current needs.

Home health-care systems can help patients leave the hospital sooner and can even prevent the need for hospitalization in the first place. However, home health-care agencies are limited by less-than-adequate reimbursement from most insurance plans. To make ends meet, the agencies have their staffs see a high number of patients per day, not allowing them to give patients the time their care truly deserves. This situation is unfortunate because home health-care systems can offer better care at lower rates and with fewer or shorter hospitalizations.

Palliative care is critically important in end-of-life planning. Oftentimes, huge amounts of resources are expended on patients at the end of life without knowing whether any of the interventions will improve the patient's health status. More important, these patients often are subjected to painful, debilitating, or needless tests or procedures that have little or often no value. Palliative care helps the patient and the patient's family come to grips with reasonable expectations, assists the caregivers to confront reality, improves the quality of care and the quality of life, and in the process saves a significant amount of money.

Hospice care is a logical and effective way of caring for those who are at the end of life. The advantages of hospice include a compassionate setting that allows death with dignity while dealing with pain and psychological and social issues. Along with caring for the patient, hospice care gives respite and relief to family and friends.

From a business perspective, vertical integration does not mean that health systems need to acquire these other businesses. It will mean, however, establishing a new set of partnerships with aligned interests to make the system work well.

Health-care reform could have, but largely did not, impact these areas of care delivery. Should the reimbursement issues be effectively addressed as part of health-care reform over time, including bundled payment systems, then we can expect the development of regional rehabilitation hospitals, sub-acute units in general hospitals, the proliferation of home health programs, and enhancements to hospice care. Bundled payment systems would also encourage the expansion of care management and network management capabilities across systems of care. We should hope this change occurs because each of these elements will lead to improved quality of care while reducing the cost of that care.

PROFESSIONAL ISSUES

The shortage of physicians, which will worsen in the coming years, will increase the need for and use of nurse practitioners, physician assistants, and others to directly assist physicians in their duties. Likewise, optometrists will do a greater degree of primary eye care, psychologists and social workers will do the majority of mental health care, and other professionals in turn will pick up the slack caused by the shortage of physicians.

In a somewhat similar manner, a nurse or other provider will be the patient's prime assistant in dealing with complex medical care protocols. The patient with heart failure or complex diabetic complications or the patient on dialysis for kidney failure must follow a difficult, challenging, and complicated care plan. The nurse coordinator can check in with the patient daily—using the phone or any number of electronic technologies, including e-mail, telemedicine, and telemonitoring—if necessary to check medication status, determine if any side effects are occurring, and generally monitor care. For the patient with heart failure, for example, learning that the patient's weight has been rising over the last few days might trigger a decision to increase a diuretic and help get the patient into better balance. This type of chronic disease management has been shown to improve the patient's quality of life overall and to reduce trips to the emergency room and admissions to the hospital. The end result is a more pleased patient and considerably reduced health-care costs.

Professional Expectations

Physicians' professional expectations will lead to substantial changes in how physicians are employed and the settings in which they work. Simply stated, their work ethic has evolved, and upon completing their training programs, physicians are less likely to enter solo or small group practices, which was the traditional pattern for more than a hundred years. Now they are more likely to want a setting where office management duties are not part of their job responsibility. They would like to have fewer on-call hours, more flexible hours, and, frankly, reduced hours. With more and more women physicians in the workforce, it is instructive to observe that women tend to enter primary care more than do men and practice somewhat differently, seeing fewer patients per hour, engaging in better communication, and focusing more on preventive care. And there is evidence that, up to a limit, more primary care physicians per population lead to better outcomes, such as life span.[1]

Physicians, especially those in primary care, have seen their income remain flat or even decline as the costs of their practice—office rent, insurance, and staff—have escalated. To compensate, they must see ever more patients, meaning longer work-days, less time per patient, or both. This situation is not good for the patient or for the physician. Those patients with complex, chronic illness do not receive the needed care coordination, which would improve care quality yet reduce costs, and none of them get the time needed for good preventive care. Displeased, doctors are turning to numerous approaches to increase their compensation, reduce their workload, or both. One is moving to retainer-based, or concierge, practices. Another is to collect an "administrative" fee from each patient each year, ostensibly to cover phone calls, e-mails, and other time commitments for which insurers do not reimburse them. Another approach is simply to refuse to accept insurance, especially Medicare, and require patients to pay out of pocket. If you have not encountered this issue yet, be aware that it is commonplace in some parts of the country and advancing rapidly in many others. These changes are truly disruptive in the way medical care is delivered.

Malpractice insurance costs are a major issue, and today many obstetricians are ending their practices because of the high cost of malpractice insurance. In 2010 I talked to a prominent neurosurgeon who had a large and busy practice in Palm Beach, Florida, but decided to retire early because his malpractice insurance had risen to the point that he felt continuing to practice was simply not worth the effort. Similarly, a superb general surgeon in private practice told me that he would like to work half time now that he has reached the age of sixty-two, but his office expenses and malpractice insurance still would cost about the same. So he either has to quit altogether or must continue working full time in order to make ends meet.

What do all these factors mean? Physicians will want to join large group prac-tices or be employed by the local hospital. They will want, expect, and demand fewer call hours, more flexible hours, and reduced hours. Basically they want to be salaried employees with the organization taking care of office issues and overhead expenses, including malpractice insurance. This arrangement would allow for an adequate fam-ily life and the ability to work part-time perhaps during the child-raising years or in the peri-retirement years. It is a major and fundamental change in physician expecta-tions and practice plans. The old idea of an independent practice, self-employment, and volunteering at the hospital has morphed into a desire for a different way of life. Alternatively, the physicians will join or develop some type of retainer-based practice so that they can have a reasonable income and a reasonable lifestyle while having the opportunity to provide superior care to their patients. Which model will prevail—a shift to the employed physician or a shift to a retainer-based practice? Probably we will see both, but certainly we can expect a shift from what we encounter in medicine today.

HOSPITAL MEDICAL STAFF ORGANIZATION

From the hospital's perspective, the medical staff will have to be organized differently because there will be more employed physicians and more specialists on the employed staff. The hospital will have to hire or at least contract with specialists such as neurosurgeons, urologists, and vascular surgeons in order to have them available to the emergency room when a patient needs their services. Most hospitals of any size will employ hospitalists to manage the patients' care while they are in the hospital, thus freeing the primary care physicians to work full time in their offices. The hospital is likely to employ pulmonologists to staff the ICUs and cardiologists to staff the coronary care unit. As a result, more physician leaders at all levels of the hospital organization will be needed to ensure a better relationship between the medical staff and the hospital executives. Gone will be the days of the hospital's so-called voluntary medical staff, or those physicians who were in private practice in the community, brought their patients to the hospital, and tended to those patients while they were in the hospital. My prediction is that with all of these changes the CEO and other senior leadership positions increasingly will be filled by physicians who demonstrate their business acumen and leadership skills, as well as their clinical care skills.

CONSUMERISM

Gone, too, will be the day when the patient is willing to be patient. As discussed in chapter 5, patients will expect rapid, excellent, and efficient care. In all likelihood, despite the reform effort providing more access to insurance, the United States will continue to have two (or more) classes of medical care, insured and less well insured or not insured at all. True, everyone will now have equivalent access to good medical care in that all will have an insurance card in their wallet. But it is already hard to get into your doctor's office today, and with 31 million more Americans wanting access to the same number of physicians, the wait times will only grow. And unless Medicaid radically increases its payment rates to doctors, don't expect too many to accept but a few such covered patients. So those who can afford it will expect a higher-level, concierge-type of care and will be willing to pay for it. As retainer-based practices become more commonplace, the remaining doctors will face greater pressures to care for those who do not opt in and are shed from their former doctor's practice as it migrates to the retainer-based format.

Consumerism, patient activism, and high costs of care already are causing another phenomenon. Some individuals go to offshore hospitals in Singapore, Thailand, and India for coronary artery bypass surgery, hip replacement, or other significant surgeries. They are finding that it is substantially cheaper to go offshore than it is to get the same major care at home. Usually the physician or surgeon trained at an American hospital and has excellent credentials. Some of these foreign institutions demonstrate that they have the same or better outcomes and quality and improved safety margins. The service is greater overall, including the pleasantness of the room, the food quality, and the courtesy of the staff. Some insurance companies will actually purchase business-class tickets for the patient and the patient's spouse or significant other to fly to the offshore hospital, pay for the hotel rooms and food, and cover the entire costs of the operation without a co-pay or deductible because the price is so much less than it is in the United States. Frankly, this better and cheaper care is not unlike other offshore "outsourcing" of professional activities that we have seen in recent years. These medical trips abroad will continue unless costs decline *and* personal service improves in the United States.

To compete, American physicians and hospitals are going to have to meet the patient's need for courtesy, service, and price/affordability along with quality and safety. It is a new challenge for our hospitals and doctors and will require a significant change in the culture found in most hospitals and doctor's offices today. Many current hospital executives will wrestle with this shift, and many physicians will resist as long as possible since in both cases it means a fundamental organizational change, from one centered around the provider (hospital, doctor, or both) to one centered on the patient. This metamorphosis has to occur, but because it is another of those disruptive or transformational changes, it will come after much struggle.

COMPLEX, CHRONIC ILLNESSES: DISCIPLINE ORIENTATION
VERSUS DISEASE APPROACH TO CARE
Another significant cultural change will be the shift from what I call treating patients with a discipline orientation versus a disease orientation. Medicine has traditionally divided itself, based on training, into internal medicine, surgery, pediatrics, obstetrics, psychiatry, and so forth. They are logical divisions because the training needed

in each discipline is quite different. At the end of the training are intensive and extensive board examinations so that the individual can demonstrate his or her competency to go out into the community and practice independently. This approach to discipline-based training, and hence the approach to care, worked well when most illnesses were acute illnesses like an appendectomy or pneumonia. The surgeon took care of the appendix and the internist took care of the pneumonia.

Multidisciplinary Teams

But what about the patient with cancer who needs surgery, then radiation therapy, then chemotherapy? The patient needs treatment by specialists trained in each of these disciplines, but from the patient's perspective, he or she is an individual person with his or her own cancer that needs to be eradicated using a team-based approach. Thus the care of complex, chronic diseases must switch from a discipline- and provider-based approach to a disease- and patient-based approach, where multidisciplinary teams work together to care for the patient. It is much better for a female patient with, say, breast cancer to be referred to a team whose members all meet her, discuss her case, and jointly offer a single plan of care, including discussion of surgery, radiation, and drug therapy along with appropriate supportive care. Now the patient will have met all of the physicians who will be handling her case in the coming months, knows what the plan is, and is assured that all three (or more) physicians agree on that plan. And, when done correctly, the three physicians along with the nurse or nurse practitioner will discuss the plan in an interactive manner with the patient, adjusting it as appropriate to fit the patient's personal needs and desires.

This approach is much different than the way it tends to work today. Currently the patient is first referred to a surgeon, who does a lumpectomy and then refers the patient to a radiation oncologist. That specialist conducts the radiation therapy and then refers the patient to a medical oncologist, who provides the adjuvant chemotherapy. The process may sound the same, but, in fact, it is a disjointed approach to care with no assurance that the three physicians generally agree on the plan of care. It is much better to bring the whole team together, to have everyone agree on a care plan, and to have one of the physicians or the nurse practitioner serve as the patient's advocate throughout the entire process and in the follow-up checks. It reduces stress, improves the quality of the outcome, and makes for a more efficient approach. Because it is well coordinated, the costs are much less. Coordinating care among providers means higher quality of care and lower costs. Most important, patients will come to expect it and demand it of their physicians.

At this point, I should mention the complementary medical approaches to care: acupuncture, massage, various mind-body techniques such as meditation or the simpler "relaxation response," nutritional counseling, exercise training, and support groups.[2] These disciplines all have their place in the modern armamentarium of treating chronic illnesses and need to be integrated fully into the team-based approach to patient care.

Here is another example of team-based care. Patients with diabetes not only have to handle the disease itself and its management, using insulin and drugs, but they have to monitor their nutrition, weight, and exercise. They need to cope with potential side effects of the diabetes, such as damage to their eyes or kidneys or the blood vessels running into the lower legs that can lead to ulcerations, infections, and even amputations. The current approach is for the patient's primary care physician to take care of the basics and to send the patient to a specialist whenever a problem arises. But the patient may need many specialists and the care is likely not well coordinated, with duplicative tests and procedures and concurrently greater costs. A much better approach is the one developed by the Boston-based Joslin Diabetes Center, which now has "franchises" across the country. The PCP refers the patient to Joslin for consultation. There the patient has a nurse as his or her coordinator and advocate, an endocrinologist to work out the specifics of diabetic drugs and insulin, an exercise physiologist to help with an exercise plan, a nutritionist to review dietary needs, an on-site ophthalmologist expert in diabetic complications of the eye, and a podiatrist to deal with foot issues. The point is that all of these professionals are available in a single location. The patient comes to one place and one place only and can go to individual, adjacent offices to see whichever specialist they need to see. If an issue or problem arises, they immediately can be referred to the appropriate specialist. The key is that these health-care providers all work as a team and bring to bear all of the different disciplines necessary to treat this complex and complicated disease for their individual patients. The result is better and more coordinated care and a more satisfied patient. It also costs much less because there is little duplication and fewer unnecessary tests or X-rays and hospitalizations. So as time goes on, more and more of these disease-based programs will emerge for the care of other complex, chronic diseases.

Marshall Steele, III, MD, is an orthopedic surgeon in Annapolis, Maryland, who did many knee and hip replacements as part of his surgical practice. He was frustrated that the medical system was not efficient, patient or provider friendly, or convenient. So he and some collaborators worked with the leadership of their hospital, Anne Arundel Medical Center, to devise a new approach to total joint replacement. Briefly, it works this way: The hospital set aside a unit with its own dedicated staff solely for total joint replacement patients. A single leader who had full responsibility and the needed authority was placed in charge, eliminating the traditional silos that exist in most hospital management systems. Instead of being focused entirely on the inputs that dominate organizations structured in departments, this new model focuses first on the outputs (outcomes) of the work from the perspective of all stakeholders. All prospective patients for the week of their surgery and postoperative care are brought in the week before to meet each other and the staff, tour the facility, and attend a class taught by a nurse-navigator who will coordinate what will transpire during their stay. They all arrive at the hospital for surgery the same day, and extra ORs are arranged for the orthopedists. After surgery the patients are put into a wellness environment outside of their hospital room. There they are brought together for eating some meals each day and for beginning physical therapy. They even return as outpatients for physical therapy together. These steps, plus many others, have markedly improved physician, nurse, and physical therapist coordination and their satisfaction while working as a multidisciplinary team, each member with his or her own expertise unleashed for the care of these patients. The patients are much more satisfied and act together as a support group. At a formal luncheon one month later, input is sought from the patients and their families, and the programs are changed to respond to their needs. The patients' length of stay is down and their complications are reduced. Important hospital-reported metrics are collected and shared with the team on easy-to-understand dashboards. Patient-reported metrics are collected on how effective the procedure was in reducing pain and on the return to desired activities.

As word got around, more and more patients, many from great distances, sought out the team. Hospital revenues rose, and the orthopedists became very busy. In the mid-2000s, Dr. Steele retired from surgery and now helps other hospitals implement this approach. But many fail. Why? Because, as Dr. Steele points out, what the program needs to succeed is a *transformational change*, but most physicians, hospital staff, and hospital management are only able to muster *incremental change*. Incrementalism where transformation is needed doesn't achieve the desired result.

This whole concept of disease versus discipline and organization around "service lines" will lead to some fairly dramatic shifts within medical organizations, another of those disruptive changes. As medicine becomes more and more disease and patient oriented, the traditional departments of medicine and surgery within a hospital will tend to be de-emphasized, and in their place will come care centers for cardiac problems, cancer, diabetes, stroke, joint replacement, and the like. A multidisciplinary team approach to such care will become much more common. As with the primary care physician, however, many practicing specialists might see this shift as a threat to their autonomy and certainly to their long-held practice patterns. Change is difficult, and as pointed out in Dr. Steele's story on joint replacement, the change needed is transformational, not incremental. While change will not come easily, it must and will occur, but not quickly.

Bundled payments, discussed further in chapters 12 and 16, will clearly assist in driving this approach to care. This financing arrangement will make it cost effective to do team-based care and use the right provider for the given situation—be that a physician of one specialization or another, a nurse practitioner, a social worker, or a pharmacist, as the case may be.

REGIONAL ECHELONS OF CARE

This whole concept of disease-oriented care as opposed to discipline-oriented care will play itself out as well in the development of regional echelons, or levels, of care. Trauma care is a good example. Maryland is recognized for having an outstanding system of trauma care, with a statewide-organized system for communication, transportation, and care of trauma victims. If an injured patient has, say, a simple broken leg, he or she will receive perfectly adequate care by a local orthopedist at the nearest hospital emergency room. But if the injury is more severe, the individual is whisked to one of the higher-level trauma centers that are scattered across the state by region. Finally, if the individual has very severe, head, or multisystem trauma, the patient is transported to the Shock Trauma Center located at the University of Maryland Medical Center in downtown Baltimore. Serious burn victims go to the Johns Hopkins Bayview Burn Center, and children with serious injuries are taken to the Johns Hopkins Children's Trauma Service. The result is the injured patient gets to definitive care within the "golden hour," or when medical treatment makes all the difference.

The Shock Trauma Center, which was built for and is devoted solely to the care of trauma patients, has a large staff whose only job is to care for trauma patients. They have become expert, and although they receive the 5 percent of patients who have suffered the most severe trauma, these patients' survival rate is better than 97 percent. The Shock Trauma Center boasts its own full-time trauma surgeons, trauma orthopedists, anesthesiologists, infectious disease physicians, intensivists, and neurosurgeons. Its large staff of nurses is trained in the various aspects of trauma care. Within the Shock Trauma facility are twelve receiving bays, six operating rooms, a recovery room, a CT scanner, an angiography suite, and an in-house clinical laboratory. Following definitive care in one of the admission bays or after surgery, a patient is transferred to one of seventy-two ICU beds divided among six nursing care units that are each focused on certain aspects of trauma care. Once the patient no longer needs intensive care, he or she is moved to one of the step-down beds and from there can be discharged either to home or to the associated rehabilitation hospital a few miles away.

The point, of course, is that a teamwork system operates from the moment the first call is received from the accident scene until the patient is discharged to home. The physicians and nurses at the Shock Trauma Center see themselves as trauma caregivers first and foremost, and as members of a particular discipline—surgery, orthopedics, neurosurgery, or medical intensivists—only secondarily.

Clearly, as with treating trauma, it would be advantageous for a few major hospitals to be well equipped with the necessary diagnostic equipment and round-the-clock staff to care for patients who have heart attacks or strokes. In the case of heart attacks, the current ideal approach is immediate transport to the cardiac catheterization laboratory, opening the diseased vessels with angioplasty, and then holding them open with a stent. Small hospitals simply do not have the equipment, the facilities, or the experienced staff to do this treatment in an expert fashion. It is clearly recognized now that transporting these patients to a fully equipped center is an improved approach to treating heart attacks, resulting in decreased mortality, decreased damage to the heart, and less chronic sequel such as heart failure. In the long term such treatment is actually cost efficient, but it requires immediate transport to the well-prepared and well-staffed hospital so that therapy can be instituted before permanent damage sets in. The same principles apply to stroke victims. Being immediately transported to a center that can begin appropriate and prompt therapy often can actually reverse any paralysis and loss of speech within minutes.

DIGITIZED MEDICAL INFORMATION

I toured a major medical center recently to look at the robots in the pharmacy and to understand how the electronic medical record worked there. I was particularly interested in the new robot that made up injectables, or the fluid bags filled with medications such as antibiotics to be given intravenously. A robot also selected pills and tablets based on bar code technology. A third robot actually delivered the medication to the individual nursing units. The robots depend on the EMR for input. It begins with the physician inserting an order that includes the drug name, dose, route, and frequency of administration. The pharmacist reviews the order and then sends it to the appropriate robot for production. This terrific system reduces errors, teaches the physician in the process, and allows the pharmacist to spend more time using his or her knowledge rather than in manual preparation activities.

I then asked to see a physician in the process of entering an order. The doctor showed me how it was done and how it helped her to avoid mistakes. Basically, she was quite complimentary of the new system. When I asked if she also found the EMR effective for writing her history and progress notes, she immediately responded, "No way. It is too cumbersome, takes much too much time, does not allow me to enter information in a logical manner. Basically it wants me to use its logic, not mine. So I just handwrite my notes." Hers was not a good recommendation, so I asked a few more physicians at different locations and heard the same response. I checked with the chief information officer (CIO) and learned that few physicians actually used the "physician documentation" part of the system, although they gave high marks to other elements such as ordering tests and reviewing results and images. Since then I have asked similar questions at multiple hospitals and always received about the same response. Clearly, there is a problem here.

Misconception 5. *Health-care costs will be reduced if we have an electronic medical record.*

President Obama has begun a $50 billion program to get the EMR into every hospital and every doctor's office. Even with this huge financial incentive, it will still take another ten years and additional huge sums of money but eventually all medical information will be in digital format. The reason for the delay is multifold. First is a serious need for interoperability among various vendors and systems. Today, it is simply not possible to easily connect one vendor system with another. This situation has arisen in part because vendors use a proprietary approach to discourage interoperability so that a purchaser, say, a hospital, will buy all of its systems from them. Fortunately, the president's EMR program calls for interoperability over the coming years.

Another big drawback today is that the various systems for documentation of physicians' and other caregivers' notes are not ideal, to say the least. Physicians for the past century have used a fairly standardized system of recording the history and physical examination and, in the hospital setting, a daily set of progress notes related to an individual patient. Most software vendors have not made this process easy and smooth in their electronic medical records, and physicians essentially rebel from using the systems for this purpose. On the one hand, frankly, they find that the current EMRs feature documentation systems that reduce rather than enhance their productivity. On the other hand, physicians admit that using the EMRs to order laboratory tests, retrieve the results of those tests, or perhaps find imaging results works effectively and efficiently. Vendors need to observe how physicians work and then design the software consistent with those practices rather than expecting physicians to change their methods to fit the new software requirements. It will not do, as one hospital CIO said to me, to say "the docs will just have to learn how to use these systems—or else." They will not use it, so far.

Physicians in a private practice setting are generally loath to buy new systems in part because they are expensive. The cost to equip a practitioners' office is estimated at about $40,000. The president's plan will greatly help to overcome this hurtle. But physicians have learned from their colleagues that these systems take months to master, and, meanwhile, their office productivity actually decreases for six months or more. At a time when physicians are terribly pushed to do more in less time, they simply cannot afford to take on a new burden that will slow them down yet again. Those doctors in settings where most of the information can be entered as "check-offs" find these systems work quite well. But the systems don't work so well for some physicians, such as internists, who need to write down extensive information from the history and physical exam.

Eventually these issues will be resolved, and then all data will be in a digital format. It will be easily accessed, easily transmitted, and secure. Electronic prescriptions will become the norm, meaning that the physician can write out the prescription on the office computer or on a handheld device and transmit it to the computer system of the patient's preferred pharmacy, where it will be checked by the pharmacist, filled, and ready for the patient when he or she arrives. In a hospital setting, a physician will use what is known as computer physician order entry (CPOE) to write out drug orders. The computer will assist in pointing out the patient's allergies and the potential interactions with other medications already in use, will know if a laboratory test needs to be ordered as part of managing the drug dosage, will help in calculating the dosage, and, where appropriate, will offer suggestions for alternative drugs that might be more effective in this particular setting. Altogether, it will lead to more effective drug prescribing and concurrently will improve safety. And with either e-prescriptions or CPOE, there is no issue about trying to read the physician's handwriting!

Even in the EMR, however, errors can still occur, and easily. Here is an example from my own experience of being referred to an ear, nose, and throat (ENT) physician for hoarseness. On the first visit he sprayed some anesthetic in my throat so I would not gag and looked at my vocal cords with a fiberoptic device that snaked down through my nose. (The remarkable instrument's diameter was about one-third the width of a soda straw, and it was very flexible. It slipped in and down easily, and he had a great view.) On my follow-up visit, he suggested that "since you don't tend to gag much," he could probably get a good enough view by simply using a mirror similar to those that dentists use. I opened my mouth, and he held the mirror in the back of my throat without touching it. I breathed through my mouth and did not gag, and he told me he got a good look. This simple procedure saved some expense since using the fiberoptic device would have meant specially sanitizing it for the next patient. He had to do the same for the mirror, but that is easier. Meanwhile, at his laptop he checked off some buttons to indicate what he had done and seen. When I left, I asked for a copy of my office visit report (as you should always do), and he printed it for me. Later, at home, I read it and found he hit a wrong check-off spot: "The view of the vocal cords was impaired by the patient's strong gag reflex." Such is the problem with computers and the electronic medical record. A message to the reader: Ask for a copy of your record after each visit to a provider and read it to be sure it has no factual errors.

Since medical images such as CT scans, MRIs, and pathology specimens will also all be digitized, they will be transmittable to any location in an instant. It means that the most experienced physician, even at a distant institution, can be called upon to review, say, a mammogram that has raised questions for the initial local reviewers or an unusual pathology specimen. This innovation obviously will save time and improve patient care at a limited increased cost. Here is an example of what happens now.

A gentleman, we will call him Otto Ehrmann, who lives in a remote area in northern Pennsylvania developed a chronic cough. He went to his primary care physician, who diagnosed bronchitis and gave him a prescription for an antibiotic. But the PCP was clearly concerned and told Mr. Ehrmann, "Come back in two weeks if the cough is not gone." Two weeks later, the patient returned unchanged. He was sent to the closest hospital, about an hour away, for a CT scan of his lungs. The result was not good; it looked like lung cancer. To definitively confirm the diagnosis he was told to come back in four weeks (!) for a needle biopsy. Why four weeks? Because the specialist at that rural hospital only did these biopsies every other Friday, and he was booked until a month later. So Mr. Ehrmann had to be patient. He returned as scheduled, and the biopsy, sent to another hospital a hundred miles away for review, confirmed lung cancer. Next he was referred to a surgical specialist in yet another distant city's academic medical center. His appointment took a few weeks to arrange, and when he met the doctor, he was told that to make a good plan for treatment he needed to get a PET scan. Although the PET center was right down the hall, it was booked for two weeks. Once the scan was done, the surgeon's office called to postpone his return appointment for a month because the surgeon would be out of town. Mrs. Ehrmann protested that was too long to wait, and the surgeon "fit in" her husband's visit in two weeks rather than four.

By chance my wife and I happened to pay a social visit to their home that day and heard his story. I called my former University of Maryland Greenebaum Cancer Center colleagues who told me that a team of a surgeon, radiation oncologist, medical oncologist, and nurse practitioner could see Mr. Ehrmann in three days' time. But he would need to bring his medical record, his CT scan, the PET scan, and the pathology report. So he had to make calls, drive to each of the hospitals, and pick up the materials. He did not pick up pictures or films but compact disks (CDs) containing his digital CT and PET scans; in other words, the records were already in digital format. Too bad these hospitals were not yet capable of sending them via the Internet to the cancer center in Baltimore. He, in effect, had to be his own FedEx or UPS carrier.

While this story is supposed to illustrate the current problems of getting information from one physician or hospital to another, it also demonstrates the remarkably poor care Mr. Ehrmann endured, waiting weeks to get the biopsy, more weeks to get the PET scan, and then another two weeks before the surgeon could see him. What Mr. Ehrmann needed was a well-coordinated, team-based approach to care, which he eventually received but certainly should have had long beforehand. This time lag happens all too often in American medicine today.

At present, hospitals do not share medical information readily. It complicates getting the appropriate care, such as when a patient is discharged from one hospital but ends up in another hospital's ER days or weeks later. Similarly, if a patient has a test at one hospital but is referred to another for a procedure, as Mr. Ehrmann's story illustrates, it is nearly impossible to send that data electronically from hospital to hospital. Instead, the patient usually has to act as a courier, picking up the information and hand delivering it to the other location. This poor arrangement takes valuable time and adds to the patient's sense of anxiety when the systems should be working to reduce patient angst. Once the electronic medical record is available on a universal basis, this difficulty should be abated. Meanwhile, hospitals that determine how to share information now, even if they do not have all the physicians' documentation materials, will find that they are benefiting patients and, in the end, their own institutions. All hospitals have invested large sums into information technology and will continue to do so into the future.

The presence of digitized medical information will mean that, finally, this information can be made available anytime, anyplace, and instantaneously. It can be placed on a chip imbedded in a card and carried in your wallet, it can be loaded onto a flash memory device similar to military dog tags, or it can be available on the Internet at a moment's notice with appropriate password protection. With my physician's new practice arrangement, I received a wallet-sized CD with all of my medical information within a few weeks of my annual exam. Now it is always with me and can be easily updated.

However the information is accessed, it is a new cultural concept for caregivers and hospitals to appreciate that the EMR is actually the patient's property. Further, each of us as patients needs to understand and recognize that the medical information is ours. This sense of ownership changes the balance of power between the caregiver or hospital and the patient. The patient no longer should be required to ask for his or her information; it should be delivered to the patient as a matter of course at the completion of every encounter. Every patient needs to understand this concept and ask (demand, if necessary) for the medical information. This shift might not be considered a disruptive change, but it is certainly a major cultural change.

TECHNOLOGY

When one considers the major innovative advances in medical devices such as pace-makers and cardiac stents for coronary artery disease or cochlear transplants for profound hearing deficiencies, it becomes apparent that engineering advances and computer sciences are a driving force. They will lead to more and more technological advances that will be of great import to medical care. There is no question that progress in basic biomedical science, pharmaceuticals, and biotechnology will continue to propel medicine, but technology will take its place as an equal driver of advances.

Technological advances clearly are expensive. Patent law protects the intellectual property that innovators develop, and the sellers seek to obtain the highest possible return on their investments. It is critical, although not only for cost reasons, that new technologies are used when appropriate and only then. But as the following discussion demonstrates, the judicious use of technology can reduce costs.

Using Social Media

Social media is new enough that no one really knows how it will become a part of medical care, but we can be sure that it will be involved and probably in a big way. Certainly it is used already for "chatting" about problems in virtual support groups. Others use it to spread the word about whether a particular doctor or other professional is any good, or at least whether that provider is pleasant, responsive, and engaging. Some people have used Facebook to get the word out that they are in need of a kidney transplant and have had quick, positive results. Others use Facebook to create groups related to their medical problem such as diabetes, amyotrophic lateral sclerosis (ALS, or Lou Gehrig's disease) and others. These sites can be used to do fundraising, share information, or publicize new research findings rapidly. As do many others, I use Facebook and Twitter to announce what I have posted on my blog. The concern is that, as with all information on the Internet, not everything posted is accurate, is FDA approved, or has been subjected to rigorous research methodology. So each of us must use social media in the most effective yet cautious manner.

Using Avatars

Doctors can develop avatars that are available to see their patients for some situations. There is some interesting experience developing in using an avatar as an addiction counselor. The patients can be part of a group therapy session without ever being seen by the other group members, and the avatar-counselor seems to lead to better attendance. Perhaps it stems from the anonymity or perhaps the convenience. Such virtual treatment approaches could be used for those living in rural areas to reduce travel time, for older patients who need frequent but easier visits to interact with their provider, and for those with physical limitations such as a recent joint replacement. While not exactly producing an avatar, newer ultrasound technology linked to image capture and graphics used in animation has allowed doctors to put on stereoscopic glasses and see a three-dimensional representation of the fetus in the womb. It serves as an invaluable tool for medical providers in assessing the fetus and gives great joy to the expectant parents to see their child as it develops in utero.

Certification Using Simulation Technologies

As the use of technology mushrooms, there will be an increased need for training and certification in the programs and apparatuses. Not only will physicians and other health-care providers need to demonstrate their competency with technology, but the technology itself also will drive new approaches to training and certification. Simulation is a good example. The classical way that a health-care provider learns a procedure is to watch an experienced physician perform that procedure, practice it under the guidance of the experienced practitioner, and then do it repeatedly until deemed competent. In the operating room, the intern generally gets to watch and perhaps hold a retractor until the end of the case, when he or she is allowed to finish putting the sutures in the patient's skin. Once deemed to be successful at that task, then the next harder task is offered on the next case and so forth. Finally after years and years of training and becoming a chief resident, the surgeon in training is allowed to serve as the operating surgeon on a case with the professor assisting but observing all the time. This system has worked for generations, but it does mean practicing on the patient before becoming competent.

As noted earlier, it is not so in the airline industry. The would-be pilot learns to fly in the simulator, and only after demonstrating both knowledge and competency through repeated exercises—including encounters with emergency landings, bad weather, and many other unforeseen circumstances—is that individual allowed into the cockpit in the copilot's position. Medicine has been way behind in developing simulation, but largely because of the advances made by the military, simulation is coming into its own in medicine. Simulators teach suturing, chest tube insertion, colonoscopy, and much more. There are simulators for learning how to hold laparoscopic equipment and use it in an efficient and effective manner while watching a monitor. In the future, surgical residents will not be allowed into the operating room to use laparoscopic equipment until proven competent on the simulator. One individual might need only a few practice sessions, while another might take many, many such practices. But the final measure will be a demonstration of competency rather than a record that "I did it seven times." In the end, simulation will decrease training time, increase competency, measure decision-making ability and technical expertise, and even quantitate the expertise of, say, a surgeon, nurse, and anesthesiologist working together as a team. An incredible advance in ensuring safety and quality care for the patient, simulation is still disruptive of the old way of learning.

Robotics

And what about robotics? Will robots take over the operating room? The currently available surgical robot, da Vinci, is used principally for prostate surgery, cardiac surgery, and some gynecological surgery. The advantages of the robot are that it never gets tired, it can lean over the operating table for long periods (humans develop back pain), it has no hand tremor, it can be programmed to avoid critical structures like a nerve or blood vessel, and it can work through much smaller incisions than the human hand is capable of doing. The bottom line is the robot can work in a precise fashion while always under the control of the surgeon who works from a console.

Nanotechnology

Nanotechnology is an exploding field in medicine for which I will offer a single example. Millions of very small tubes are created at the nanoparticle level, which is incredibly small (nano means one billionth of a meter). These tubules can be constructed in such a fashion that they will serve three functions at once. By attaching a compound to the tubules, such as a monoclonal antibody, and injecting them into a patient's vein, the tubules can find a target, say, a lung cancer cell. Attach to the tubules an agent that can be visualized on an imaging device, and it will be possible to see on the CT scan or MRI exactly where the tubules have found the lung cancer cells. This location might be in the lung, but it might also be in local nodes or in distant organs, demonstrating that the cancer has spread, or metastasized. Finally, it would be possible to attach to the tubules a drug or a radioactive particle that can destroy the target, in this case the lung cancer cell, without affecting other cells. Hence the nanoparticle carries out three functions at once: finding the target, visualizing the target, and destroying the target. This transformational technology will be another major advance in medical care.

EVIDENCE-BASED CARE

Care providers are well educated and well trained, and the vast majority work hard to remain up to date. Nevertheless, best practices do not necessarily reach practitioners in a timely fashion as opposed to the community's general belief to the contrary (see misconception 4). The result is that they do change their practices but slowly, even when the data on newer or different approaches is compelling and based on strong evidence from well-conducted clinical trials. Providers, however, need to use the best evidence-based information available while caring for patients.

Increasingly, professional societies are offering guidelines for the care of specific diseases or situations based on strong evidence. They update these guidelines regularly as new information becomes available and is properly tested. In chapter 15 I will review the concept of a Federal Health Board that, if properly designed and executed, could accelerate these efforts and ensure that all providers are able to access the current best practices easily.

MAJOR REDESIGN OF MEDICAL CARE DELIVERY

In essence, the various changes I have discussed mean an overhaul of the medical delivery system in America. The various forces, or drivers, include demographic changes, more chronic illnesses, greater need for preventive care, professional shortages, changes in professional career expectation, and major advances in the medical care armamentarium. It needs to all come together in a new system of care.

Today, and tomorrow, our ability to predict the onset of disease, to diagnose an illness, and to treat a patient effectively has risen dramatically. Meanwhile, we need to accept the reality that not all frontline providers need to be physicians, that not all provider-patient encounters need to be face to face anymore, that quality and safety must be improved, that the results of evidence-based studies can markedly improve care yet help us avoid unneeded or ineffective care, and that providers must follow protocols and checklists in order to give the best care.

One of the important first steps in reorganizing care delivery is for care providers to become patient centric rather than provider centric and to develop teams with a disease-based focus. These teams, or individual providers where appropriate, need to rely on standardized approaches to diagnosis and treatment that are varied for the patient's specific needs. Hospitals, clinics, and even doctor's offices need to be reorganized so that the infrastructure serves the needs of the providers' new approach to patient care. These redesigns of the care delivery system will not come easily, but they ultimately will occur in order to match the patients' needs and demands, the expectation to provide greater quality and safety, and the requirement for keeping care cost effective.[3]

Academic Medical Centers

On the one hand, academic medical centers (AMCs) by their very nature have great disadvantages in dealing with the trends into the future. They are large, cumbersome, and extremely slow to make decisions. They have multiple missions, including research and education, which are not always critical to the patient's best interest for care provision. On the other hand, they are well positioned to improve outcomes as new technologies, devices, approaches, and medicine—genomics, stem cells, and immunologic approaches along with nanomedicine technologies—are developed, since they are tested in the academic medical centers first. Then they will be evaluated and refined there, and the new knowledge will be dispersed into the community medical setting. Similarly, eMedicine (telemedicine, ePrescriptions, etc.) began in the academic medical centers and will continue its march into the community. Another element that benefits the AMCs is that the hospital and the physicians are, or at least can be, organizationally aligned.[4] This arrangement differs from the community setting where the physicians working in a community hospital are, to a large degree, in private practice and are not in the employ of the hospital.[5] At the AMC the opportunity is there for the school, its faculty physicians, and the hospital to agree on an approach to the "new medicine." In short, if nimble, the AMCs can benefit from the future trends.

AMCs can also pioneer the development of team-based, multidisciplinary coordinated care using the disease-patient approach rather than the discipline orientation. Centers devoted specifically to treating trauma, cancer, stroke, and diabetes are all examples. They improve patient care and safety while reducing waste and costs. But they do not conform to the usual discipline-based structure and practice of the medical school, the hospital, or the faculty practice plan. The idea of a trauma-centered practice plan that includes surgery, orthopedics, internal medicine, and anesthesia is anathema to the traditional departments, yet it is essential to the effective functioning of the disease- and patient-based center.

If AMCs can pull together, they can lead the nation with new, more effective, and less expensive approaches to the care of complex, chronic illness. With prudent coordination of that care, they can also achieve better quality, safer outcomes, and reduced costs.

AMCs are also the ideal setting to train medical students and residents in how a team works, how to flatten the hierarchy, and how to interact and debate effectively. They can also develop the needed medical leaders to advance medicine into this new age.

I hope they are up to the task.

Design of Health-Care Delivery Facilities

Here are a few comments on how hospitals and other facilities will be designed as a result of the trends we have discussed. To be effective and efficient, their design will begin with an understanding of what patients and their families want rather than simply what the providers want. For example, the facilities will take great efforts to promote respect for patients' preferences, dignity, and values. The design will consider the need for physical comfort and effective pain management and take into account the requirements for emotional support and the control of fear and anxiety. The needs of family members, long ignored in design planning, will become integral. Design parameters will recognize what has been repeatedly emphasized in this book; that is, most hospitalized patients will have chronic, not acute, conditions and often multiple chronic illnesses, and many will be older with all the differing needs of the geriatric population. The design will incorporate the needs to ensure a safe environment and include approaches to assist in safety measures. Given the high risk for hospital-acquired infection, the new hospital will be designed with techniques to reduce the spread of infection as much as possible. Since they will use more and more technology, the design of hospitals will need to take into account that technology changes considerably over short time frames. Finally, the design of hospitals must consider managing costs, not only during the construction, but over the life of the building. Here then are a few of the new design principles.

All patients will be in single rooms. This layout is important for ensuring privacy and rest, and it is critical for preventing the spread of infection from patient to patient. The rooms will also have plenty of space for family members or friends to visit if the patient wishes. Rooms will also be designed to be "acuity adjustable," meaning that the room can be readily converted from a regular room to an ICU room based on the patient's needs; this adaptation will reduce transfers to another area of the hospital as much as possible. Hospitals will be designed with a healing approach, incorporating the use of light, the visualization of nature, materials that reduce noise, and good interior design principles. Instead of medical and surgical wings, they will feature specific care centers for cancer, cardiac problems, diabetes, and so forth.

Doctors' offices will be congregated near where they work—that is, in the centers—rather than being aggregated around their training discipline, such as medicine and surgery. Nurses will have work pods near the patients rather than at distant nurses' stations. They will have good lines of sight to observe patients. The staff will use extensive information technology to assist their work and their documentation. Patients and their families will also access important information with this technology. These are but a few of the new design concepts that are important for the future.

SUMMARY OF THE MEDICAL CARE DELIVERY OF THE FUTURE

Unrelated to what health-care reform will create, I believe it is clear that certain changes in medical care delivery can be fairly well predicted. As these changes occur, many will be incremental, whereas others will be truly disruptive or transformational. Yet it still is and probably will be true that, not withstanding common misperceptions, many advances will not reach the actual practice of medicine quickly. Some, as laparoscopic surgery did twenty years ago, gained traction remarkably quickly; but others, such as simulation today, seem to take much longer than would be ideal. And the notion that the EMR will be ubiquitous in a few years is simply not likely.

Unfortunately, nothing on the horizon from the insurers or the government reforms suggests that there will be an emphasis on health promotion and disease prevention. Indeed, we seem to be losing ground on that issue at a substantial rate. The one bright spot is that many primary care physicians have decided either to bill the patient directly for services and not accept insurance or to switch to retainer-based practices. In both of these models, the PCP can reduce the number of patients under care and thereby give the remaining patients the time needed for preventive services and for chronic illness care coordination.

PART III
THE COST OF MEDICAL CARE
IN AMERICA

The costs of medical care are rising rapidly and consume a remarkably large and growing part of our incomes. Little has been said about the true reasons for these rising expenditures, but they are neither difficult to understand nor insurmountable. That said, it will take a Herculean effort to actually create the mechanisms that will hold the rate of increase at a manageable level while overcoming many entrenched interests. But if we do, and there is no good reason not to do so, then everyone will save money, including the government. The additional dollars can pay for the insurance that the less fortunate desperately need. As I will explain, improving the quality of care delivery will reduce costs. In my opinion, when legislators developed the Affordable Health Care Act, they should have focused first on improving care, which in turn would have reduced costs to the individual, businesses, and state and federal governments and thereby allowed the extra dollars to enhance access for all. But it is not too late for Washington to address costs through quality and safety improvements.

Health-Care Financing:
Basic Concepts

Misconception: *Universal coverage for all Americans will reduce costs.*

Stomach ulcers are a fairly common problem. As noted in chapter 4, it turns out that most cases are caused by a bacterium called *Helicobacter pylori* (*H. pylori*). It was discovered in 1982 that this bacteria is able to live in the stomach despite all that acid, invade the wall of the stomach, and create the ulcerous condition. But being a bacterium, scientists also discovered that it could be treated and cured with antibiotics. After much trial and error, a number of regimens have been found to be most effective. A typical one involves taking two different antibiotics, clarithromycin and amoxicillin, twice a day for two weeks. These antibiotics are more effective if they are taken with one of the proton pump inhibitors (PPIs), or acid suppressors. It is critical that the patient takes both the antibiotics and the PPI twice a day without fail for fourteen days, or the cure rate decreases substantially. Because this regimen includes a fair number of pills, it can become a bit confusing for some patients. So the makers of the PPI called Prevacid assembled a nicely designed package called Prevpac that contains the two antibiotics and the PPI, and each dose is clearly labeled: "Monday morning's pills," "Monday evening's pills," "Tuesday morning's pills," and so on. It makes it easier for the patient to remember exactly what to take and when. Frankly, it is a good idea.

When an acquaintance was found to have an ulcer caused by *H. pylori* and his internist gave him a prescription for Prevpac, it cost about $350 at the pharmacy. Prevacid, one of the drugs in the Prevpac, was until very recently on patent; hence, its price was still very high. Given that this combination of drugs cures the ulcer, it is not an unreasonable price to pay to eliminate a disease that in the past had been chronic and impossible to cure, often reduced one's quality of life, and frequently necessitated surgery.

But here's the catch: If you have commercial insurance with a prescription benefit, you probably only pay a $15 co-pay for the drugs. Not bad, from your perspective. Interestingly, if you chose to buy the three drugs separately, the total cost would be about $250. But even though it costs less and you are quite competent to remember to take the required pills every morning and evening for two weeks, you probably do not want this deal, because for you the price is higher. Using your insurance, you would have three $15 co-pays, or pay a total of $45, and the insurance would pay the balance.

If instead one substituted the over-the-counter (OTC) drug Prilosec for the Prevacid, it would bring the price down further, to about $100. The effectiveness, the safety, and the cure rate would be the same, but the profit would not be; so there is no package arrangement for these three drugs at the lower price tag. Instead, again you would have to buy the individual medications and remember to take them as directed—certainly not an impossible task. Multiply the savings of about $250 by the number of individuals with *H. pylori*–causing stomach ulcerations, and you will save big money nationally. But once again our incentive system is badly flawed and discourages this option. Your personal total cost is now $60: two $15 co-pays for the antibiotics and $30 for the Prilosec (insurance doesn't cover over-the-counter medications). So you will opt for the most expensive package for the "system" but the least expensive for you. And in all probability your physician will be aware of this financial issue and so recommend that you use the Prevpac.

Many believe that universal coverage for all Americans will reduce costs. Unfortunately, that is not the case; indeed, it will create substantial added expenditures. While we should be ashamed that America is the only country in the developed world that does not ensure for everyone at least basic medical care coverage, offering coverage to all will cost someone—you and me—in taxes. It is true that having access to a physician for basic medical care will mean fewer visits to the emergency room, fewer hospitalizations, and better overall health for the individual. It will reduce the overall cost of care, but there are still substantial real costs for getting medical care to the 31 million additional people envisioned in the reform bill. To think otherwise is to ignore reality.

Tackling the real cost issues and the societal issues of our behaviors will be difficult no matter what and particularly difficult for elected officials, who certainly do not want to annoy either the industries that support their campaigns or the voters who will need to make significant changes in their lifestyles. This reluctance is unfortunate because it needs to be done, and without a strong federal example from the bully pulpit along with incentives for change, change that is so critically needed will not simply materialize.

IMPLICATIONS FOR EMPLOYEES' WAGES

Our current system of health care is not economically viable. Businesses and the U.S. government both carry a large burden of the health-care costs for Americans. Businesses simply cannot afford it, and this situation is exacerbated because we are part of a worldwide economy. If our costs of doing business are too high and are reflected in our products' prices, some other country will produce them less expensively, taking jobs and revenue overseas. Large corporations that had promised health-care benefits to its retirees found that they could no longer afford them and have off-loaded that charge to others. In the automobile manufacturers' case, it was moved to the union. Smaller businesses, especially those in the service industry, often find that they simply cannot afford health insurance and do not provide it to their employees. We often do not stop to realize that if our employers are spending more on health insurance, then they will spend less on our salaries. The result is that higher expenditures for health insurance in the past decade have resulted in lower wage and salary increases than would otherwise have been the case.

The government cannot afford the health-care burden either. There is a limit to the government's ability to tax the populace. Today Medicare and Medicaid consume 4 percent of the gross domestic product, and that share will continue to rise if no changes are instituted to control rising costs. Some suggest that businesses should take on the responsibility of health-care costs for all employees no matter what, and others suggest that it should be totally shifted to government. On the one hand, if businesses accept or are forced to insure everyone, then there will be a decrease in profitability, a loss of jobs, and higher costs for products and services. America will become less competitive in the worldwide economy. On the other hand, if the burden is placed on government, then it will inevitably lead to an increase in taxes. In short, there is no "free lunch." Indeed, the Medicare tax has been increased as a result of reform. The only way to solve this predicament is to slow the rise of medical care expenditures or, much more difficult, actually reduce current costs. So it is absolutely essential that a comprehensive approach to health-care cost management be a part of reform into the future.

Many would say that even more money is needed in order to give health-care coverage to those who are not insured today. For sure, it will be expensive. If the cost per person insured today is about $7,500 to $8,000 per year, then that number multiplied by the 31 million uninsured now expected to get coverage is more than $200 billion per year. With no other changes, that money will have to come from our taxes. I would argue instead that the dollars currently in the system need to be reallocated in a more effective and productive fashion so that we can give health-care coverage to everyone while providing good-quality, efficient, affordable, well-coordinated medical care. In one step, if everyone had a primary care physician they saw on a regular basis who was incentivized to offer real preventive care and coordinate chronic care, then substantial cost savings would result from keeping them healthy and from keeping those with chronic illnesses out of emergency rooms and avoiding unnecessary procedures, drugs, and hospital admissions. Effective coordination of care between acute care and post-acute care—such as skilled nursing facilities, inpatient and outpatient rehabilitation facilities, home health and hospice agencies, and long-term acute care—can reduce hospital readmissions, thereby reducing spending and greatly improving patient experiences. But accomplishing these goals, and the other needed changes, especially a change to ensure well-coordinated care, will require major system-wide change. For example, there are not enough PCPs today, and if they are to give quality care to a smaller number of patients each (I recommend about 500 patients per physician), we will need either many more PCPs or many more additional providers. As another example, in order to provide seamless patient care across the post-acute continuum, Medicare should review its policies and remove the regulatory and financial barriers to collaboration and integration that currently exist.

Most of us with employer-based or government-sponsored insurance have a limited understanding of the economics of our coverage. What we do know, if we are among the 87 percent who have medical coverage, is that it seems expensive, doesn't seem to cover what we need, isn't there when we need it the most, and has all sorts of exclusions. The insurer's administration is hard to contact, mired in bureaucracy, seemingly hell-bent on denying us benefits we thought we had, and, if not, then determined to send us pages and pages of documents that are difficult to read and interpret.

Most people do not know what is being spent on their behalf, or the total insurance bill. Most would be surprised to learn that a business pays, on average, about $13,000 for a family medical policy and nearly $7,500 for an individual. The premium has increased nearly 140 percent over the last decade. If that rate persists—and there is no current reason to think otherwise—then in ten more years, the insurance cost per family will be more than $30,000 per year. Today, if employed by a business that offers insurance, the employee pays about 27 percent of that total. That would be about $3,500 per year now and a whopping $8,400 in 2019. What's more, to try to slow the rising rates of premiums, companies expect you to accept higher deductibles and co-pays, to use only generic drugs, and to obtain prior approvals for nonemergent visits to specialists, tests, procedures, or elective surgeries.

——— DRIVERS OF CHANGE
- Total cost of health care in the United States: 17 percent of GDP and rising rapidly
- Rising health-care costs: about 10 percent per year
- Increased dissatisfaction with current health-care financing
- Increasing and large numbers of uninsured and underinsured
- Health-care reform, a political reality

THE TOTAL COST OF INSURANCE

Insurance premiums keep going up each year. You know that when your employer says that you must pay more when the annual sign-up time comes around each year. You pay a larger percentage as well. In 2000 the average cost of employer-sponsored medical insurance for a family was about $6,438. In 2010, a decade later, it had more than doubled to $13,370.[1] And of that amount, you paid $3,997. For that money, you get much less in return, for most plans have morphed from a conventional plan, where you could go to any doctor or hospital with a small deductible, to some type of managed care plan with a network of doctors and hospitals that you must choose from, a larger deductible, and more co-pays.

If you obtain your health policy directly from an insurer, you may have decided to go with an "underwritten" policy. In this instance, the carrier checks your health status, and if everything is OK, it then agrees to accept you in the plan. The rate is much lower, perhaps about $5,000 per year, and comes with a high deductible, usually $1,000 or more. With this plan you can have a health savings account, which lets you put in pretax dollars and then use them for your deductibles, co-pays, drugs, and so forth. It can represent a substantial savings. The government has approved this concept with the idea that you will be a more cost-conscious buyer of medical care since you will have more invested in the process.

Most of us think of Medicare as being free, or paid by the federal government. But in actuality you pay 1.45 percent of your earned income—and your employer does the same, for a total of 2.9 percent—into the Medicare Trust Fund every year that you work. Add it up, and it's a great deal of money. Those funds are used for Medicare Part A, which is basically meant to cover hospital care. Part B covers doctor bills and is split equally between you and the government, which pays its portion out of general tax revenues. Currently the individual's Part B base rate is a little more than $100 per month and is deducted from your Social Security payments. Medicare A and B pay about half of allowed bills, so most retired individuals buy a supplemental, or "Medigap," policy from a commercial insurer. It's one more expense that costs about $1,500 per year or more. And then there is Medicare Part D, the drug coverage. Rates vary by insurer, but the average across the country in 2008 was about $30 per month or $360 per year. (We found that our cost in the local BlueCross/Blue Shield Part D plan was initially $32 per month and had risen to $77 per month in 2010. We switched to a high-deductible policy in 2010, and it's down to $35 per month.) Add all of these fees, and you will be paying at least $3,000 annually for your total Medicare coverage and twice that for you and your spouse combined.

The point is that whether our employer or the government provides the coverage, we individuals still incur substantial expenses. Since most insurance does not cover everything, we have additional expenses. Most important for our discussion here, few of us recognize the full amount that is being paid for our medical insurance, because we never see it. In the case of employer-based insurance, the rising total cost severely limits wage increases and will do so more and more in the future. Consider Mr. Miller, earning $50,000 per year working for a firm that provides insurance for its employees. He is expected to pay about $4,000 for family coverage. What he does not realize is that the total policy premium is about $14,000, so the company is paying the balance, or $10,000. If he does realize it, he is probably thankful that the company pays for it. Come time for his annual review and hoped-for salary increase, the company says it can add 3 percent to its wage pool. That money could represent a $1,500 increase for Mr. Miller, but the company also reports that it must now pay 10 percent more for the medical insurance, meaning that it now costs the company $15,400 per year. Mr. Miller must now pay $4,400 or $400 more, and the company picks up the other $1,000, which cuts the increased funding pool by $1,000. Mr. Miller can only get a $500 raise rather than the $1,500 raise. As benefit costs go up, wage increases will be inversely affected. So it behooves us to understand the implications of a rising medical care insurance premium because even if we do not pay for it directly, we pay indirectly in lost wages.

EXPENDITURES FOR MEDICAL CARE

Health-care costs in the United States consume more than 17 percent of the GDP, and this share is rising rapidly. They represented about 5 percent of the GDP in 1960 and 12 percent in 1990. Medical cost inflation is about 6–10 percent per year, which is much greater than general inflation. The outlays for health insurance have risen 119 percent since 1999 while the average workers' earnings rose 34 percent and inflation rose 29 percent. Insurance companies' administrative costs, which are basically the difference between premiums received and benefits paid, have risen sharply per person covered, from $217 in 1995 to $453 in 2006. Not surprising, health-care employment as a percent of nonfarm employment has risen from about 7.5 percent in 1990 to about 13 percent today. Although it may be difficult to find a physician, especially a PCP, when you need one, especially in rural and poor urban areas, the number of doctors per 100,000 persons has actually risen at a fairly steady rate, from 146 in 1970 to 319 in 2007. Most of this increase is in specialists. But physician incomes on an inflation-adjusted basis have gone down over the past decade. In 2003, primary care physicians earned a net income of $146,000, which is down 10 percent since 1995 after adjusting for inflation. Surgical specialists collected a net income of $271,000, down 8 percent since 1995 after adjusting for inflation. During the same time frame, incomes for professional, technical, and specialty workers in the private sector rose 8 percent, inflation adjusted.[2] With specialists earning more than generalists, most medical school graduates opt for specialization.

For the year 2007, health-care spending rose 6.1 percent to a total of $2.2 trillion, which represents $7,421 per American.[3] General inflation in 2007 was 2.8 percent.

It is interesting to note that about 48 percent of all medical care spending is for 5 percent of the population. And about 73 percent goes for only 15 percent of individuals.[4] Just as Willie Sutton robbed banks because "that's where the money is," in the medical care system, we need to focus on those with chronic illnesses again because that is where the money is. Who are these individuals who use 15 percent of all medical care spending? They are mostly those people who have complex chronic illnesses: heart failure, diabetes with complications, cancer, multiple sclerosis, chronic lung disease, kidney failure, and other serious illnesses. This statistic reminds us that complex, chronic illness, which affects only some of us, accounts for the lion's share of expenses. If you develop one of these diseases, even with good insurance you may find yourself in difficult financial straits because insurance only covers so much. Reform needs specifically to address the care of those with these complex illnesses to control cost escalation.

THE LIMITS OF INSURANCE COVERAGE

Views diverge on what medical care insurance should cover. One recommends comprehensive coverage from prevention to annual exams to routine care to diagnostic tests and procedures all the way to catastrophic hospitalization or the use of expensive drugs. This coverage means essentially "prepaid" medical care, albeit often with some co-pays and deductibles. It includes prescription coverage for essentially all medications whether for lifestyle needs—birth control, stress-induced erectile dysfunction, acid blockers for those who eat highly spiced foods, and so on—or for actual illness. The other end of the spectrum advocates coverage only for the more catastrophic events, leaving the individual to pay out of pocket for prevention, annual visits, routine care, and most prescriptions. The latter description was what most people with insurance had a few decades ago, but the trend over time has been toward making insurance coverage more and more comprehensive, particularly within large corporations, with or without union contracts. (And once we have a benefit, we don't want to lose it; so our political leaders avoid tackling it.) A middle-ground approach might be for insurance to cover an annual examination with appropriate screening and preventive care counseling along with catastrophic coverage kicking in after meeting a sizable deductible.

Here was one of the critical questions as the country debated health-care reform: Do we subsidize the uninsured and the underinsured to obtain a full-fledged comprehensive policy, a policy that only covers catastrophic events, or a policy that assists with basic, preventive, and catastrophic care? It needed to be discussed directly but never was to any extent. The final result in the Affordable Health Care Act is a plan that covers basic prevention services with no co-pays or deductibles, limited high-deductible plans, and essentially everyone gets complete, prepaid medical care with every policy sold commercially and with Medicare. To me this solution represents keeping the old formula and ensuring everyone has access, but it will not stem the tide of rising costs as it would have if it went back to being real insurance—that is, providing coverage for catastrophic needs with a high deductible. When we have a high deductible, we pay attention, we ask our doctor more questions, and we become appropriately skeptical of suggestions for tests and procedures. We also become the best agents to prevent and eliminate fraud. Being more skeptical or recommendations and being more alert to abuses would lower the costs of care substantially.

CONTROLLING COSTS

Politicians and pundits often suggest that we can reduce costs by "hammering" the hospitals, the drug companies, physicians, the insurers, or the lawyers. Essentially Medicare does that by setting its reimbursement schedule at a level slightly below current costs for hospitals and physicians. And insurers do it by setting their rates for reimbursement to physicians and hospitals below costs as well. The concept is to let the providers figure out a way to reduce their costs. The problem is that they do not individually hold the levers needed to accomplish much. Price controls rarely work in medicine or anywhere else in the economy. I would emphasize that this price setting is not a strategy; instead, it is a short-term tactical maneuver to hold the line as much as possible and for as long as possible. It's obviously not working, since medical care costs continue to rise rapidly. A new approach is clearly needed.

Certainly the hospitals, doctors, drug manufacturers, and others bear some responsibility at the margin, but the real focus on reducing medical costs cannot be laid upon any of them. The truth is that there are no "bad guys." Certainly the drug and device manufacturers want to sell their products, the hospitals want an adequate income to allow for reinvestment in facilities and new technologies, and physicians, just as all of us, want to earn more. Those desires are natural. So what needs to be done? We need better systems of care—care that is coordinated, evidence based, and transparent to the patient—and more attention to quality and safety. To make this improvement happen, the system needs to be changed to include meaningful incentives for physicians to offer preventive care and care coordination, for physicians to become primary care providers instead of specialists, and for all of us to lead a healthier lifestyle. We need a focus on preventive care. We also need an aggressive approach to change the cultural factors that lead to poor personal behaviors, which in turn result in trauma and severe, lifelong chronic disease.

We also have excess regulations, many of which add costs but little value. That in turn creates waste, so regulations must balance their efforts at reducing fraud against the costs they add to the system.

Medical care costs are rising primarily as a result of a few key drivers. Interestingly, we mostly read and hear about the less important drivers, causing us to misunderstand the role of new technologies in medical care's cost escalation. As noted previously, we have a large and increasing population of individuals beset with complex, chronic conditions that tend to last a lifetime and are inherently expensive to treat, but we spend far more than necessary on treatments that often do not meet the expectations for quality. These individuals consume the bulk of all medical expenditures in large part because their poorly coordinated care results in excesses: more visits to their physicians, specialty physician referrals, lab tests, imaging, procedures, and hospitalizations. Further, care varies widely for the same condition from region to region and even among providers from the same hospital. These complex, chronic diseases are the result of two factors—aging, which leaves people inherently more susceptible to disease, and engaging in behaviors adverse to good health. Diabetes with complications, heart failure, chronic lung disease, and many cancers are directly attributable to poor nutrition, obesity, lack of exercise, stress, and smoking. Once developed, these illnesses tend to persist for the remainder of one's life so that the expenditures for care continue until death. Steven Burd, the CEO of Safeway, notes that industry has found 70 percent of their health-care costs can be attributed to people's behaviors. About 74 percent of these expenditures go to treat four diseases: cardiovascular disease, cancer, diabetes and obesity[5]—yet the vast majority of these illnesses are preventable.[6]

Add to this mix the unusual way we pay for medical care, that is, via a third-party payer. Because we individuals do not typically contract with our medical providers as we do with other service providers (for example, our lawyer, accountant, architect, or carpenter), our doctor "works" for the insurer. To a large degree, we are not the insurer's customers, either; our employer or the government is the true customer. This arrangement creates an aberrant economic system in which the patient, who is neither the customer nor the client of the doctor or the insurance company, is at a disadvantage when confronting a medical problem.

Two recent reports help to define the issues of rising health-care costs. The consulting firm McKinsey and Company prepared a report in December 2008 on why American health care costs more than that in other developed countries.[7] In a brief summary of the report's findings McKinsey compared American health-care expenditures to those of thirteen peer countries from the Organization for Economic Co-operation and Development and from that data developed a measure called estimated spending according to wealth (ESAW). This measure adjusts health-care spending relative to a country's per capita GDP. In 2006, the year with the most recent and complete data, the United States spent $2.1 trillion (about $6,800 per person) for health care, or about $650 billion more than the OECD peer countries did, even after adjusting for per capita GDP, or wealth. It amounts to about $1,600 additional spending per American per year for health care. Where was this money spent? Two-thirds of the spending above what the peer group expended—let's call it excess—paid for outpatient care, including physician visits, outpatient procedures, same-day hospital care, and community diagnostic centers such as radiology.

The McKinsey data is consistent with the results of researchers at Dartmouth Medical School who have been evaluating variations in the costs and patterns of care across the United States. They suggest that where there are more specialists and where there is more "capacity"—that is, the total combination of available doctors, nurses, clinics, hospitals, technologies, and so on—they will get used more often and drive up the total cost of care.[8] The finding sounds similar to the adage of "build it and they will come."

In a recent analysis of Medicare data from 2001–2005, the Dartmouth investigators looked at the last two years of life for Medicare recipients with complex, chronic diseases such as heart failure, kidney failure, and dementia. They picked those two years of life because they account for a large proportion of all Medicare expenditures. They found vastly different costs owing to a wide variation in the use of services such as specialists, stays in the intensive care units, hospital stays, and so on. This finding related directly to the local medical care capacity. Where there was more capacity, there was more use and therefore higher expenditures. On average these patients each accounted for about $46,000 of expenditures by Medicare during those last two years of life. In states with high capacity, such as New Jersey, the average expenditures per patient were $59,000 while in an area where capacity is relatively low, like North Dakota, the average expenditure was $33,000. It is certainly a wide difference, yet they could find no significant disparity in the quality of care or patient outcomes.

So why are costs so high and rising so fast? Are we getting better care? More care? And why is it that our medical costs are so high compared to that of other developed countries? Based on my interviews with practitioners and business leaders nationwide and on my own experiences as a clinician and health-care executive, here are the principal reasons why health-care costs are high and rising so fast:

- Shift from acute care to chronic care
- Poorly coordinated care that also varies by geographic region
- New technologies
- Personal behaviors
- Aging population
- Inadequate quality and safety
- Higher drug costs
- Emphasis on prescribing drugs instead of lifestyle changes
- Using brand-name instead of generic drugs
- Broken malpractice system
- Unnecessary tests and procedures.
- Failure to accept death when it is inevitable
- Broken insurance system
- Lack of primary care physicians or their equivalents
- Inadequate methods for transferring critical medical information
- Inadequate patient education/transparency

Chapters 8–14 will address these issues and questions in some detail. Then I will propose an approach to improving the quality of care while concurrently reducing its costs.

The Real Reason Why Our Health-Care Costs Keep Going Up

Misconception: *Health-care costs are rising because of avarice and greed or unregulated "bad guys," including drug and technology companies, doctors, hospitals, malpractice lawyers, and third-party payers, or insurers.*

Henry is a sixty-nine-year-old widower, living alone in a small town in Ohio about sixty miles from the nearest metropolitan area. He has a small pension and has health-care coverage through Medicare and a Medigap policy. He was recently hospitalized in the intensive care unit with a serious urinary tract infection that had spread to his kidneys (pyelonephritis) and to his bloodstream (septicemia) for which he was given potent antibiotics by vein. After a stormy few days, he recovered.

A week later Henry called me and asked for some advice. He was taking twenty-three different prescription drugs, some once, some twice, and some three times per day along with one by shot monthly. He was not certain why many of them had been prescribed and asked if I thought he needed them all. I responded that, being four hundred miles away, I could not be his doctor, but I would review the list and offer some questions he could ask his physician. He sent me the list. I reordered it by category: two for heart failure (he did not know that he had heart failure), two for diabetes, three for high blood pressure, one to lower his cholesterol, a monthly shot of testosterone for impotence, one to shrink his prostate (it was felt that an enlarged prostate had been a predisposition to his urinary tract infection), one for depression, one to finish treating his kidney infection, and nine other prescription medications.

I learned that he did not have a primary care physician; rather, Henry went to four different doctors, each of whom treated different issues—none of them had all of his information and they did not communicate with each other. Whenever one of them checked his blood pressure, it would be elevated, so that doctor would either add a drug or increase the dosage. He told me that when he went to the local drugstore and checked his blood pressure, it was always normal. I told him that he might have "white-coat hypertension," meaning it was only high in the doctor's office. Perhaps if Henry took his regular readings to the doctor, the physician would take him off one or more of these drugs. Besides, two of the three had a known side effect of impotency. I also noted that he was on one drug to shrink his prostate yet the shot of testosterone might well be causing some of his prostate enlargement.

Henry's story represents much of what is not working in the delivery of medical care today. His four complex, chronic illnesses—heart failure, diabetes, hypertension, and depression—all require attention and care coordination, preferably by a single PCP who knows his home and social setting as well as his direct medical issues. The blood pressure medication story is another example. Further, he was getting much too many drugs that he did not need and had probably become impotent as a result. Rather than looking for the cause, a doctor gave him another drug (testosterone) that probably had no value but was likely enlarging his prostate. As a result, he had developed an infection that had almost killed him. Finally, all these drugs were expensive, both for him and for his Medicare Part D insurance plan.

Heart failure and diabetes together consume more than half of our health-care dollars, yet no one adequately monitored Henry's care; rather he was getting one drug after another without attention to what else was happening. This lack of care coordination is a prime example of why the health-care costs are so high yet its quality is still so low.

My first suggestion was that Henry needed a primary care physician, one to call his own. He learned that a young doctor he had met at a nearby hospital would be setting up a private practice near his town, so Henry became one of his first patients. A few months later he told me that he was taking seven medicines, felt better, and was saving a great deal of money.

Henry still has four serious chronic conditions. But with a single physician serving as an orchestrator rather than simply as an intervener, one who actually pays attention to Henry's social and home life, Henry has better quality medical care and a much higher quality of life. Also, he is spending less money—both his money and that from Medicare, Medigap, and Medicare Part D. In short, his coordinated care plan is a win-win for all concerned.

OVERVIEW OF APPROACH

As policymakers approached the issues of health-care reform, they needed to decide where to start. With access? With care quality? With costs? I firmly believe that the correct starting point was and still should be with care quality. Better quality, including improved safety, will mean reduced not greater costs, and the savings can then be applied, in part, to improved access while giving everyone—individuals, businesses, and government—a lower burden to fund. Henry's story is a good example of improved quality leading to both better health and lower costs.

We hear all the time about the bad guys who are making enormous profits from our disease misfortunes, but these stories are merely stories. Sure, there is some truth at their margins, but the list at the end of chapter 7 details why medical costs have escalated and why the total cost of medicine is so high. So how can we reduce the costs of health care or at least slow the rate of their rise? We have a natural tendency to believe that if costs are reduced, then quality will be reduced as well. I hope to convince you that the opposite is the case: Improving the quality of care will be the best way to lower expenditures. We can have better care while spending considerably less money. To improve quality while controlling health-care costs will require a coordinated, integrated, and comprehensive approach. No single approach will solve the entire problem, and for sure we will need to address the various barriers to implementation, barriers that are intense and will not be maneuvered easily. Henry's story is a good example of how simple, inexpensive steps can markedly enhance quality and concurrently reduce costs. His situation is not an exception; it is all too common. So let's address the issues one by one while recognizing that they make up a total picture.

To improve care quality while reducing costs, five approaches stand out as most important. The first four are coordinating the care of disease, developing strong health maintenance and disease prevention programs with an emphasis on improving our personal lifestyle behaviors, addressing the impact of aging, and paying much more attention to safety. To accomplish this work will require the fifth step, reforming insurance so that it incentivizes appropriate behaviors by the patient, physician, and hospital and reconnects the doctor and the patient as vendor and customer. Three of these are discussed in this chapter; safety and insurance in later chapters.

IMPROVING QUALITY AND REDUCING COSTS WITH CARE COORDINATION

To improve care and reduce expenditures, we must coordinate the care of those with chronic diseases. One approach is for more organized systems of care. To a large extent, this idea is counter to how doctors and hospitals function today, where everyone is autonomous and functions independently. This is not to say that physicians are not well educated and trained—they are. Nor does it mean that they do not try to keep up with the advances in medicine—they do. But it does mean that the most effective, evidence-based medicine is often not appreciated and certainly not followed; that care is not coordinated; and that patients end up getting unneeded diagnostic tests and procedures, excessive elective surgeries, and hospitalizations that could have and should have been avoided. A real change in the way medicine is practiced, especially in the way care is coordinated, will reduce health-care costs particularly for that small minority of patients who generate the vast majority of total health-care expenditures.

Some well-known clinics, such as Mayo, Geisinger, Marshfield, Dean, and others, provide good, coordinated care today. Some common characteristics allow them to be effective. First, they are organized as large groups of physicians with a shared sense of professionalism within the group. Physician members are those who prefer, or at least accept, the concept of a managed organization. The physicians are salaried but are still expected to cover their expenses. The doctors understand that they will probably earn less than those in a private practice setting, but in return they have fewer hassles, they do not have to grow a patient base because the organization already has one when they are recruited, and they will practice in a single hospital that is generally managed in a way to make their work smoother. These group practices usually have good information systems that allow a patient to be referred to another group member the same day, and the patient's information moves with the patient.

In this system, the entire patient experience is organized around the patient, not the group practice. The work is allocated broadly among those who can best accomplish it, from primary care physician to specialist physician, nurse to nurse practitioner, clinical pharmacist, and so on. They make outstanding use of other technologies to enhance care, such as the telephone, e-mail, and other electronic methodologies, in addition to an electronic medical record. Most have large groups of capitated patients, meaning that it is in the physicians' best interest to manage the cost of care along with the quality of care. And if they manage the capitated patients appropriately, they inevitably handle all patients in the same manner. It results in well-coordinated care that is of excellent quality yet is less expensive.

The idea that America needs more integrated care systems is now new. In 1933 the Committee on the Costs of Medical Care (then about 4 percent of GDP) recommended that "medical service should be more largely furnished by groups of physicians and related practitioners organized so as to maintain high standards of care and retain the personal relations between patients and physicians."[1] The opinion was based on evidence that group practices provided high-quality care in a more efficient manner than solo practitioners did. This issue is even more relevant today given the multidisciplinary, team-based care that patients with complex, chronic illnesses require. Large groups can effectively accept capitation and distribute the income proportionately to the providers involved. This system is difficult to accommodate in solo practices or small group practices although the development of larger "virtual" groups could solve some of the associated problems.

We need to have many more physicians functioning in a similar manner, whether or not they belong to one of these large, well-known groups or clinics. One of the most obvious and most relevant is to assure that PCPs take on the responsibility for care coordination of their patients with chronic illnesses. To do so means serving fewer patients more intensively, as I discuss in detail in chapter 13.

How can we move toward a more coordinated system given the makeup of our provider population and its training today? Here are some tested approaches.

Disease Management

The concept of disease management means a single physician, usually a PCP but in some instances a specialist, acts as the orchestrator for all the caregivers, probably assisted by a nurse or nurse practitioner, especially for patients with the most complex diseases. The nurse works with the patient to follow the often complicated care protocols outlined by the various physicians. Telemedicine can assist here, as it can reduce visits to the provider and the emergency room and admissions to the hospital. Evolved disease management can improve the quality of care and as a result the patient's quality of life. Medicare sponsored a few demonstration projects to determine if a nurse coordinator could improve care and reduce costs through education and monitoring.[2] A few clear messages emerged. First, the care coordination needs to be frequent. Second, the coordinator must collaborate closely with the patient's physician; they need to work as a team, not simply interacting briefly as they administer care.[3]

Medicare also has established the Medicare Advantage program, also known as Part C, which allows groups that are similar to a health management organization to accept a capitated payment for the total care of Medicare recipients. In addition to the usual Medicare benefits, they also provide good preventive care, including vision and hearing screening, cholesterol checks, and vaccines, and many supply drugs at a reduced rate. Currently these programs receive an extra 14 percent payment from Medicare, apparently to help these organizations get established. Not surprising, this subsidy has become a political issue, and it will be rescinded over time as a result of the reform legislation. But Congress needs to be careful when determining its cuts. The extra 14 percent of funds might not all be necessary, but the program's concept is excellent and should not be undermined.

Some Medicare Advantage organizations limit their membership and only accept those with one or more of a defined set of complex, chronic conditions, such as heart failure or end-stage kidney disease. These plans work on the principle that the organization will actively coordinate the patient's care. Care coordination plus preventive care improves quality while reducing costs. With the reduced costs, the organization makes a profit, so it is incentivized to be effective. But these programs succeed only if they are able to get the physicians, hospitals, and all of the caregivers working together as a team. Simply appointing a coordinator is not adequate.

Life Management Programs

One can combine the elements of a wellness program (discussed later in this chapter) and disease management program into a life management program. The concept here is to intervene with good preventive care while the individual is still healthy and to give coordinated care to those with chronic illness. The Erickson Retirement Communities (ERC) have been pioneers in this regard. By way of background, the company's basic goal was to improve the quality of life for its residents. So ERC built in nutrition, exercise, and other programs for the residents who live in campus-like settings. Yet it found that its biggest failure from the retirees' perspective was medical management. As a pilot program, ERC hired a physician who initially spent about thirty minutes for each patient's visit. As word got around, more residents signed up for his care. Eventually he had to cut back until he was seeing each patient for about ten to twelve minutes per visit. Again the residents were not satisfied. ERC hired additional full-time physicians and paid them enough in salary over what Medicare paid so that they could afford to take the needed time with each patient. It quickly became apparent that the residents liked this approach, but it meant each physician could only see about four hundred or so patients rather than the national trend of about twelve hundred to fifteen hundred for a primary care doctor. It cost more up front, but Erickson found that the number of hospitalizations for this group declined by about 50 percent, suggesting that good coordination of care not only increased satisfaction and quality but also effectively reduced costs. The reduction benefited Medicare, but Erickson still had the extra expense of the added physicians to make the program work.

Erickson approached Medicare and petitioned for a demonstration project. After being turned down for some years, Medicare agreed, in part because ERC had computerized records of all care and Medicare thought that some useful data might be generated by a demonstration project. To date, more than four thousand retirees in multiple retirement communities joined ERC's Medicare Advantage program. The results again confirmed the value of good care coordination, a computerized medical record, and orchestration of chronic care by a PCP who could spend adequate time with each patient. At one retirement center, for example, inpatient hospital days dropped from a national average of 2,096 per thousand Medicare enrollees per year to less than 500. And since these retirement communities generally have older residents, the average age is higher than for Medicare patients nationally. Adjusting the data for age meant that it was equivalent to only about 200 hospital days per thousand residents per year. Another helpful metric is an unplanned return to the hospital shortly after discharge. The national rate for Medicare recipients is near 25 percent, an incredible number, but the Erickson plan has kept these to 10 percent. (Frankly, having one-quarter of Medicare patients end up with an unplanned return to the hospital within thirty days of discharge is outrageous and another testimony to the inadequacy of care coordination for those with chronic illnesses.)

One key to ERC's success was having the PCP serve as the orchestrator of all the patient's specialists, ensuring that the patient's medications were appropriate, not mutually adverse, and in the correct dosage for a geriatric person. The primary care physician also attends the resident when hospitalized, bringing the patient's EMR to the hospital on the doctor's laptop. ERC found that if the patients were cared for only by the hospital-based hospitalist, the tendency was for the acute problem to be well managed but for other issues to get out of control, leading to longer stays and various complications. As a result of the PCP's involvement, ERC's program can ensure that the residents continue to get appropriate care for all of their needs and not only for the particular problem that sent them to the hospital. Nursing care coordinators are involved in tandem with the primary care physician, who has the needed time with each patient. They conduct regularly scheduled programs of health management. As with employer-based wellness programs, ERC offers behavior modification courses but also introduces specific programs for monitoring, coaching, and preventing specific high-risk diseases. Non-physician providers are used extensively, which helps to keep the costs down and the contact level high.

In short ERC's plan is a wellness program with behavior modification, a close care management program, and an aggressive disease management program of complex, chronic diseases from their onset rather than when they become problematic later on, all rolled into one. But Medicare was reluctant for some time to grant the plan continuing status. John Erickson, the founder, comments that Medicare is "not nimble. It sees itself as a funding manager, not a medical management organization." The result is that Medicare has difficulty accepting or even encouraging the type of approach begun at the Erickson Retirement Communities. Medicare administrators seemed focused on whether a broad segment of the population is benefiting equally—the retirement community is self selected and middle class, not a county or other political subdivision—rather than endorsing model approaches for high-quality care, with high patient satisfaction and a much-reduced cost.[4]

In short, what is needed is the development of accountable care systems—actual, virtual, or combined—that address care coordination of complex illness in a manner that increases positive outcomes while controlling costs:

- Incentives from both Medicare and commercial insurers to encourage the development of care coordination systems that use the primary care physician (or a specialist, in certain circumstances) as an orchestrator along with ancillary staff and other nonphysician health-care providers to maintain a high level of personal contact with each patient
- Changing from the current volume-based payment systems to a system that pays for coordinated care of complex, chronic illness
- Payment systems that recognize the value of e-medicine, namely, e-mail, telemedicine, e-prescribing, and so on

CHRONIC DISEASE PREVENTION TO REDUCE COSTS
Not only do we need to better manage the care of chronic illnesses when they occur but, better yet, to prevent these diseases from occurring. This will markedly reduce the continuing rise of medical expenditures.

Personal Behaviors
An important reason for cost escalation has to do with our own personal behaviors, which reflect the nature of our culture. The costs of our negative behaviors are actu-

ally more important in the long term than those associated with our overuse and misuse of technologies. Many Americans are overweight—one-third are overweight and another third are obese—do not exercise enough, have poor nutrition, and are highly stressed. And it gets worse each year. We even find that children's physical activity progressively declines from about three hours per day at age nine to less than an hour by age fifteen. This inactivity will correlate to obesity beginning in adolescence.[5] Twenty percent of us still smoke tobacco. These factors are some of the major reasons that medical costs will rise in the future. They lead not only to diabetes, heart disease, arthritis exacerbated by obesity, and shortened life spans but also to enormous medical bills.

Our government needs to encourage good health, regardless of the economic interests that such a program will affect, and we individuals need to accept true responsibility for our actions. First, it will mean eating less fatty food, less red meat, less whole milk and less cheese on our pizza, and fewer sodas (and everything else made with high fructose corn syrup) and prepared and take-out meals. It should also mean preparing more meals at home and incorporating more whole grains (whole wheat, brown rice, oatmeal) into our diets and in the cereals sold in supermarkets. We need to shop the periphery of the supermarket and leave the aisles with all the prepared foods alone. (Here is a simple rule of thumb: If you must buy a prepared or packaged food, look at the ingredients label. If it has more than five, put it back on the shelf. If it contains ingredients you never heard of or cannot pronounce, put it back. And if it lists sugar as the first ingredient, unless it is candy, put it back.) Next, we must stop smoking and encourage teenagers not to pick up the habit or they will incur the wrath of lung cancer, heart disease, lung diseases, and others illnesses in the future. Then we must accept that weight gain is a function of the number of calories consumed minus the number expended by exercise. It's a simple equation, but apparently we find the answer so difficult that we instead try all sorts of diets that ultimately don't work but cost money and frustration. Finally, chronic stress is a cofactor in heart disease, back pain, gastrointestinal disorders, and many others. We need to adjust our lifestyles to compensate.

We tend to think of most deaths as being from heart disease, cancer, or stroke, but another way to think about it is to consider what the underlying causes of those illnesses were. As noted in chapter 2, 40 percent of all deaths can be attributed to behaviors that could be modified. The leading causes of death in the United States in 2000 were from tobacco use, poor diet and physical inactivity, alcohol consumption, infections, toxic agents, motor vehicle accidents, firearms, sexual behaviors, and illicit drug use.[6] Most of these are behavior-related illnesses.

Wellness Programs

Wellness programs are based on the concept of helping an individual modify his or her behavior to prevent future illness. It is a good and tested approach; moreover, improved health means not only fewer illnesses but also decreased absenteeism and greater worker productivity. Most wellness programs are based at the workplace, where incentives are instituted so that employees will find it easier to modify their behaviors. Corporations offer specific programs for smoking cessation, weight reduction, nutrition, stress management, and exercise. Although not required to join, employees are given an incentive to join the program by having, for example, their share of the cost of health insurance reduced as a result of participation. Some companies have realized major cost reductions in health-care expenses. General Mills reported a 20 percent reduction in health-care costs after implementing its wellness programs. As of 2010 Safeway had held total all-inclusive per-employee healthcare costs at 2005 levels whereas most other large American companies have seen a cumulative increase of about 50 percent over the same time period.[7] As noted in chapter 7, the grocery chain based its program on two insights. First, 70 percent of all medical costs are the result of adverse behaviors, such as smoking, overeating, and lack of exercise. Second, 74 percent of all health-care costs are related to cardiovascular disease, cancer, diabetes, and obesity, conditions that are, for the most part, preventable with behavior modifications.

As another example of using financial incentives to encourage healthy lifestyles, a large, multinational U.S.-based company agreed to conduct the following trial: 878 employees were randomly assigned to receive information about smoking cessation programs with or without a financial incentive. The incentive was $100 to take and complete the program, with $250 more for cessation at six months and an additional $400 for cessation at twelve months. Those participants who received the incentives were more likely to join a cessation program (15 percent versus 5 percent), complete a program (11 percent versus 3 percent), and be tobacco free at six months (21 percent versus 12 percent) and at one year (15 percent versus 5 percent).

Clearly, wellness programs work. Basically, they offer people incentives to take responsibility for their own health. They link rights and responsibilities together.

Behavior Modification

Some would argue that affecting behaviors is not the role of the health-care system. I disagree; the doctor wields plenty of influence to help patients modify their behavior. With incentives for doctors and patients alike, major inroads could be made on smoking, diet, weight, and exercise, all of which are at the top of the list. Changing behaviors is where we can have the greatest impact at the lowest cost.

If 40 percent of deaths are related to behaviors that could be changed and 74 percent of expenditures are related to only four complex, chronic diseases that can be largely prevented, then these behaviors are worth addressing. Tobacco is the most important behaviorally related cause of disease and death; we need to find ways to stop smoking and to discourage teenagers from starting to smoke. About a third of Americans smoked in the mid-1970s. Thirty years later, the proportion had fallen to about 20 percent, but it is still much too high. But nicotine is addictive, perhaps more addictive than illicit drugs are. Withdrawing, and therefore quitting, is hard to do. We need role models. Here, President Obama could be our best hope of becoming an example and encouraging others finally to kick the smoking habit.

We also need to transform our sedentary lifestyle. Exercise, nutrition, stress reduction, and weight management are critical. We need a national program to teach and encourage Americans to maintain a healthy weight and eat a nutritious diet. First Lady Michelle Obama is taking a leadership role in encouraging better nutrition with fresh foods. Controlling one's weight is difficult, as the continuous wave of new diet books attest. People always have excuses, but in the end, to be healthy, we simply cannot have a population that is one-third overweight with another third obese. Using body mass index (BMI) as a measure, we have gone from an adult average of about 25 (normal range is 18–24.9) in the mid-1970s to about 28 in the mid-2000s. The more notable increase occurred in those who are obese (obese is BMI of 30–34.9, morbidly obese is greater than 35).

Good dietary habits, along with exercising, need to begin in childhood and include preparing food from basic ingredients rather than buying prepared foods; using whole grains, lean meat, and vegetables; and avoiding fatty foods and processed foods. Again, if you read the label and cannot understand what each ingredient is, then you shouldn't eat it. We need to encourage families to eat dinners together, slowly enough to enjoy the food and to appreciate what Mom or Dad prepared. With some appreciation, Mom or Dad might be inspired to do it again the next day and not call out for pizza. I have been fortunate to have a wife who for more than forty-eight years, while attending college and graduate school, child rearing, and working, has always found time to prepare meals from good and healthy ingredients. As a result, we've enjoyed pleasant, nutritious mealtimes over the years. Cooking for the family really did not take her that much time, and she enjoyed the creativity along with the pleasure it produced. Now our daughter, a mother herself, writes a blog about the high-quality foods she prepares, ones that are allergen-free for the benefit of her children, who had multiple food allergies in their early years.[8]

We already know certain types of programs work to help people change their lifestyles: the workplace wellness programs with monetary incentives for behavior modification such as the one introduced at Safeway (chapter 7); the Healthy Howard program, which includes incentives to live a healthy life and overcome personal barriers to success (see chapter 3); and the Erickson Retirement Communities' approach to wellness. These and other similar programs can have a major impact on our overall health. They need to be endorsed and replicated.

Screening Tests

Screening tests for blood pressure, cholesterol, cervical cancer, and some other diseases are clearly cost effective if not downright inexpensive, especially when considered in the context of the diseases prevented and the lives saved.

Far too many of us do not get simple tests for our blood pressure and cholesterol levels or simple cancer screens like the Pap test. These screening tests can detect abnormalities that, if addressed early with relatively inexpensive approaches, can prevent serious, costly illness from occurring at a later date.

A friend called to say that he had gone to see his physician one day when he did not feel well only to find the physician was out of town. His nurse took the gentleman's blood pressure and found it to be quite high. She informed the patient but did not otherwise give any advice. Later that morning he called me because he was concerned about his blood pressure, his coworkers said that his speech sounded strange, and he was developing a headache. I had him ask a colleague to bring him to the ER, where he was promptly admitted with an impending stroke. Immediate therapy brought down his blood pressure, but it required a stay in the neurological ICU for a number of days and in the hospital for a few more days after that. The moral of my story is, of course, that if his high blood pressure had been diagnosed, probably years before, and appropriately treated, not only would he have avoided an admission and great stress, but the health-care system also would have saved tens of thousands of dollars.

Some screening tests—for example, a colonoscopy—are more expensive per test, but if they are preformed for those at risk, the cost in terms of disease prevented or life prolonged is reasonable. Some preventive measures actually offer economic value, that is, actually create a savings. These steps include smoking cessation programs, childhood immunizations, and aspirin to help ward off coronary artery complications. At the same time, it is important to realize that some preventive services are not of great economic value, although for the individual patient found afflicted it may seem beneficial. For example, it makes no sense to do colonoscopies for individuals younger than fifty years old unless they have a genetic risk of colon cancer; then it can potentially save their lives. Similarly, there may be specific individuals for whom reducing low-density lipoproteins (LDL), or "bad cholesterol," below 100 is valuable, but it is of limited economic value if pursued for most people.[9]

The new guidelines for breast cancer screening and cervical cancer screening were designed with these sorts of considerations in mind. We now know that the human papillomavirus causes most cases of cervical cancer. The new vaccine against HPV will therefore prevent these cancers if given before the individual is infected. And for those who have had multiple negative annual screenings, the current guidelines suggest that Pap screening every three years is satisfactory, and for this group, no screening is necessary in women after the age of sixty-five. In 2009 the U.S. Preventive Services Task Force also changed the guidelines for breast cancer screening. It no longer recommends teaching breast self-examination, suggests that most women do not need to start mammography screening before age fifty (instead of the former baseline year of forty), and concludes that biennial mammography is satisfactory for women at normal risk. Finally, the task force found that the evidence is unclear whether the benefit to risk ratio is sufficient to continue screening after age seventy.

Some highly medically effective and cost-effective measures nevertheless take a long time to impact disease prevalence. It will be no simple matter to change Americans' personal behaviors regarding poor nutrition that, in turn, stem from socioeconomic issues, the availability of low-priced fast foods, and the switch from nutrient-based to commodity-based agriculture that imparts much less nutrient value to the calories derived.[10] And the impact of changed behaviors will take many years to reduce the disease burden on society. That said, the return on investment, both economically and in terms of better health and longer lives, for changing behaviors will be of major consequence some years down the road. But this potential is of little consequence to political leaders who feel the need to achieve short-term benefits in time for the next election cycle, especially when reforms will undoubtedly require addressing issues that well-funded lobbyists will aggressively resist. But it can be done, as the Safeway example demonstrates. Appropriate incentives for healthy, responsible living can result in fairly immediate results: better health, lower costs, and more productivity.

Public Health Measures

In the late nineteenth century, the big advances in health came as a result of disease prevention. Sanitation with sewer systems, safe water systems, and pasteurization of milk all had a profound impact in reducing some of the most common and serious diseases of the time, such as dysentery, typhoid fever, and tuberculosis. Then came vaccines for diphtheria, pertussis (whooping cough), and tetanus (lock jaw), and once again a major reduction in disease occurred. Proper handling of foods including safe canning practices was also important. These advances were all about preventing rather than treating disease.

Vaccines

We need to ensure that each of us and our children get the appropriate vaccinations. Because of various ill-founded concerns, such as the fully disproved possible development of autism in our children, all too many parents do not get their children vaccinated against the common childhood illnesses. As a result, for example, measles outbreaks occur when the disease, unwittingly imported from another country, travels through communities of children who have not had their measles vaccinations.[11] We forget that this childhood illness can be severe and that elsewhere in the world children are dying in large numbers from diseases like measles. Likewise, adults do not get their influenza shots each year despite the fact that thousands die from flu each year. I venture to say that most of you readers over the age of sixty have not had your pneumococcal pneumonia or your shingles vaccine. As I discussed in *The Future of Medicine*, vaccines not only prevent infections, but I also believe eventually research will produce vaccines that will prevent or treat some of our major chronic diseases, such as atherosclerosis, Alzheimer's, some cancers, and autoimmune diseases such as type I diabetes mellitus, rheumatoid arthritis, and lupus erythematosus.

These major advances for medical care, however, will only occur if the pharmaceutical industry feels reasonably protected from unnecessary, ill-founded, and disruptive lawsuits.

Vaccines are the most cost-effective means of reducing disease; we need to use them to the maximum extent. They will ultimately save us all a great deal of money in illness care and, more important, give us better health.

INCENTIVES

To encourage people to change their personal behaviors, obtain basic vaccines, and get appropriate screenings, we need incentives. One approach would be to incentivize citizens with insurance premiums. Insurers could offer reduced premiums for those who do not smoke, for those who obtain vaccinations and appropriate screening tests, and for those who regularly exercise and maintain a reasonable weight. This proposal is not unlike what the auto insurance industry already offers—that is, reductions for maintaining a good driving record and for taking a driver's education program. I do want to be clear that this suggestion is not akin to refusing to insure someone for a predisposing condition; it is only to incentivize each of us to lead a healthier lifestyle.

We can also encourage good health via an appropriate school lunch program that feeds our children and grandchildren a nutritious lunch without junk food. We can have much better truth in advertising and continue to improve the labeling of processed foods so that we know what we are buying in a supermarket. More communities should follow the lead of New York City to eliminate trans fats from fast-food restaurants. Simply posting calorie counts, which restaurants resist, helps us to understand the implications of our decisions before we make them. This is more of "nudge" than an "incentive" and we still might make the wrong decision from a health perspective, but at least we will know what the decision means in terms of calories, fats, and so on.

One of the best ways to encourage changes in personal behaviors is to create workplace wellness programs with clear and meaningful incentives. Safeway's and General Mills' programs create effective incentives to lower the employees' cost of health care substantially in return for their addressing adverse behaviors.

In sum, an intense focus on our personal responsibility and behaviors offers the greatest opportunity to improve health and reduce disease. Behavior improvements can markedly reduce illness and premature deaths, which is, of course, the ultimate goal, but at the same time they also can reduce the cost of health care. As part of that initiative we all need incentives through our insurance premiums to encourage good behavior; healthier school lunch programs; and better truth in advertising and information about the foods we eat, such as posting calorie counts in restaurants. Workplace, church-sponsored, or retirement community wellness programs can help us adjust our behaviors and effect real change. Meanwhile, we need to expand our public health initiatives and markedly encourage the development of new and exciting vaccines that can have a positive impact on reducing illness.

MAINTAINING HEALTH WHILE AGING WILL REDUCE COSTS

America, as with all developed countries, has an aging population, meaning that a greater percentage of the population is elderly. As discussed previously, the elderly suffer from the majority of complex, chronic diseases. As we get older, most of our organs and muscle mass decline at a fairly fixed rate of about 1 percent per year beginning at about age thirty to thirty-five. But exercise will slow the rate of decline. Restated, our bodies (and our brains) are meant to be used regularly.

One measure of monitoring our bodies' decline is bone mineral density. This term refers to measuring the strength of our bones. During infancy, childhood, and adolescence, we steadily build up the strength of our bones though our diet, especially with the intake of calcium and vitamin D and by exercise. By the time we are about twenty years old, our bones have become as strong as they are going to become. If our diet was deficient or we did not exercise enough to encourage proper bone development, then our bones will always be weaker than they could have been had we followed a really good diet and exercise regimen. Since bones strengthen with exercise, we can start life as an adult with very strong bones. As we lose about 1 percent of our bone mineral density per year after age thirty or so, eventually we reach a point where our bones become fragile, and some suffer from osteoporosis.

In our aging population, women have a greater tendency for broken hips than do men. The broken hip is a problem in and of it self, but it often translates into other serious problems as well such as pneumonia, lack of mobility, being house bound, losing social interactions, and more. This prevalence in women is for two reasons. First, during menopause that 1 percent rate of bone density decline increases by a few percentage points per year for three to five years and then flattens out again. Thus, women have lost quite a bit more bone mineral density than have men at that point. In addition, women tend to live longer and, as a result, in the later years of life are at risk for a fracture. What can be done? First, although for most of us it is too late to effect change, we need to start in childhood a nutritious diet and regular, aggressive exercise so that by the age of twenty people will have very strong bones. It will give them a higher point from which to start the 1 percent annual loss in bone density. It follows that by starting at a higher point, it will take longer to reach a stage where the risk for fracture occurs. Second, we can still exercise during adulthood. Bones respond to exercise, so a good exercise program of simply walking twenty to thirty minutes per day will help keep our bones strong and slow that loss of bone mineral density. Add to this routine a good diet and some calcium and vitamin D supplements, and we will keep strong bones a while longer. Of course, some drugs are now available, but they really should be used only by people who have truly attempted to maintain their bone strength with exercise, diet, and calcium and vitamin D supplements yet still find their bone mineral density has fallen too low. Then, if necessary, drugs can be a major help, but they do have potentially significant side effects.

Finally as we reach older age and are at risk for a fracture, it is important to do those simple things that will keep us from falling. We can continue our exercise regimen, work on balance exercises, get rid of throw rugs that we might slip on, be sure to have grip bars in the bathroom and rails on the staircase, and be extremely careful on ice and snow. And we can get our vision checked to be sure our glasses are appropriate and use a walking stick if needed to improve balance—safety needs to override pride.

While there is no fountain of youth, we can with proper care and maintenance slow down this inexorable process of loss in our bodies. Just as we can curb bone mineral density loss, so, too, with exercise and a good diet can we retard the process of losing muscle, lung, and heart function. While we can preserve our bodily functions as long as possible with simple lifestyle changes, we can slow the decline of our brains as well. Exercise sends blood to the brain, and evidence suggests that we also should engage in good mental exercises, such as playing chess as opposed to watching TV. Similarly, exercising the brain has been shown to slow down memory loss and may delay the onset of dementia. Add good nutrition, regular exercise, and maintenance of normal weight, and watch what happens to one's health.

There is no question that we can enjoy good health if we maintain a healthy lifestyle into our later years. Lifestyle requirements need not cost much and should be encouraged with financial and other incentives, for good health means much lower expenditures for medical care.

— 9 —

The High Cost of Drugs and Technologies

Misconception: *New technologies are major culprits in rising health-care costs.*

You had probably never heard of restless leg syndrome before you first saw it mentioned in an ad on television. It is a syndrome where for no apparent reason, often when you are lying in bed, your legs seem to need to move, sometimes with a twitch, sometimes only a slight motion. It is annoying and can annoy your partner in bed as well. It stops as soon as you fall asleep or as soon as you get up and move about. I have to admit that I had never even heard about it until I read an article about it in a medical journal. As soon as I read it, I realized that I had it myself to a mild degree. My experience is enough to be annoying sometimes but not enough to seek treatment. But now a drug is available, and the pharmaceutical firm, launching a nationwide ad campaign, would like you to be aware of it. Its message, simply stated, is if you have restless leg syndrome, the pharmaceutical company would like you to go to your physician and encourage him or her to give you a prescription for its drug. For the drug company it is a great way to increase sales, especially for a syndrome that most people have not heard of before. But every drug has its side effects, so if your problem is not really significant, it is probably best not to be taking a pill. There are those who will greatly benefit from this drug, but I certainly am not going to ask my doctor to prescribe it.

NEW TECHNOLOGIES AND PHARMACEUTICALS

The pharmaceutical, biotechnology, and medical device and medical equipment companies have been extremely effective at innovations that have created major benefits for medical care. The cost of new devices, such as pacemakers, defibrillators, stents, ventricular assist devices, insulin pumps, laparoscopic surgical instruments, and so forth, are high. Patent policy allows for the company to recoup its research and development expenses, and this practice has fueled innovation. The problem, of course, comes with the use of a drug or a device that is not needed or indicated or that is not really superior to an older and cheaper model or drug.

For example, almost everyone has had heartburn at some time. On television, you will see advertised one or more drugs for treating heartburn. The ads want you to think that serious, chronic acid reflux esophagitis is a problem for nearly everyone; that the drug advertised is certainly better than any others that are available; and that you should hurry to your physician to get a prescription. The facts are somewhat different. Reflux is common, and in most people, it can be handled with making simple lifestyle changes. Putting the head of the bed up on blocks so that the acid "runs downhill" and stays in the stomach can make a big difference. So can waiting two to three hours after dinner before going to bed so that the food in the stomach has been digested and passed on. So, too, can reducing alcohol and caffeine consumption since they increase acid output. Then there are effective yet less expensive medications, such as over-the-counter antacids. But all these suggestions require making a change on our individual parts, and it is much easier to go to the doctor and ask for the pill.

Now certainly some people do have serious chronic reflux and need one of these new medications that reduce acid production in the stomach. There are two types of these drugs. The ones that were introduced first have brand names such as Tagamet (cimetidine) and Zantac (ranitidine). They proved to be extremely effective in treating patients with ulcers when they first became available in the late 1970s and early 1980s. But then a new class of drugs called proton pump inhibitors became available, the first of which was marketed as Prilosec. (Others are Nexium, Protonix, and Prevacid.) Tagamet, Zantac, and Prilosec are now off patent and are available over the counter, while Nexium and Protonix are still on patent and available only by prescription. Clearly the ads are meant to encourage you to ask your physician for a prescription for one of the patented drugs. Is this step necessary? The straightforward answer is absolutely not. While the patented drugs are excellent, effective, and extremely safe, they cost about $150 for a two weeks' supply. The OTC Prilosec is an almost identical drug that has an equal degree of effectiveness and an equal degree of safety. You can pick up a two-week supply at a supermarket for about $28. In fairness, a few patients with severe chronic reflux find that the prescription drugs work better or are more effective than are the over-the-counter versions. But these cases are few and far between.

Here's a catch. As I noted in chapter 7, if you have a prescription plan as part of your employer-sponsored insurance and buy Prilosec over the counter, you will pay for it, all $28, with your own money. If you get a prescription drug from your physician, you probably pay about $10 to $15 as a co-pay and the insurance pays the rest. It is actually therefore cheaper for you to get a prescription from your physician to treat your heartburn than it is to have your physician recommend taking OTC Prilosec. Such is the craziness of our current reimbursement system in medicine. And of course there is never a "free lunch," because this substantial sum contributes to keeping insurance premiums high.

Although not the principle reason for rising costs, new technologies can certainly be a cost culprit as well. Consider the example of laparoscopic gall balder removal, which has increased expenditures nationwide. As a new technology, overall, it improved costs, patients' quality of life, and patients' outcomes. But now gall bladder surgery is being done more often than in the past, presumably because the surgery is less invasive; the recuperation time is quite quick, meaning less time away from work; and the overall discomfort is low. So an individual might opt for getting the surgery done that he or she might have procrastinated about in the past. Or the physician might encourage it, saying, "You really ought to get this done because it will solve the problem and you will be fit as a fiddle afterward."

Consider the cell phone as an analogy. In the late 1990s, they were expensive and few people used them. Today, now that they are inexpensive, everyone has one, using them almost exclusively and for purposes not even dreamed of ten years ago. The overall number of dollars being spent for cell phone and wireless technology has gone up dramatically.

Misconception: *If my doctor prescribes a drug, orders a test, or suggests a medical device, I should go with that recommendation.*

At a minimum you should question your doctor about any test, imaging, procedure, or drug that is recommended. Ask why: "Will the test make a difference in my treatment? Is there a less expensive drug or will lifestyle modifications do just as well?" And if a procedure is recommended, you might want to get a second opinion. Always do your homework—ask lots of questions.

REDUCING INAPPROPRIATE OR UNNECESSARY USE
OF NEW TECHNOLOGIES

The most critical step to controlling the inappropriate use of new drugs and technologies is to incentivize primary care physicians to be thorough and to deliver good care coordination. This measure would reduce a vast array of visits to specialists, tests, imaging, procedures, and even hospitalizations. Much of the overuse and inappropriate use of medical care stems from physicians not taking the time to do a careful history and examination. The answer is to create monetary incentives for PCPs to reduce their practice size of about twelve hundred to fifteen hundred patients to about five hundred patients, thus leaving enough time for each patient on each visit. But this reduced patient load means each visit must cost more and be paid either by insurers or out of our own pockets. Another approach is to encourage the development of more clinic-type, large group practices that accept capitation, or prepaid care, and are committed to both preventive care and chronic disease care coordination.

We need some limits on drug and device advertising. Of course, perspectives differ on this issue, but drug advertising on television and radio is largely inappropriate. The pharmaceutical firms will argue that they are simply educating the public so that in turn people can ask their physicians about a new drug or a new device and see if it fits their circumstances. Such is the case with restless leg syndrome in the story that started this chapter. Sure, patients need to be informed so that they can ask their doctor appropriate questions, but most of this advertising is all about priming folks to request a prescription, not really to ask for advice. So I would recommend increased Food and Drug Administration oversight to ensure more appropriate drug advertising and stricter regulations to prevent implying that a branded drug is superior to a generic drug or that a drug is needed when lifestyle changes should be taken first.

A third area that needs to be addressed is the lack of interoperability of devices and information technology. Since many devices do not interconnect, a hospital must either buy all of the devices from one company, thereby reducing competition and increasing prices, or purchase some additional systems to create the interconnections necessary. The same goes for information technology, as discussed previously. It is critical that national standards be established and that all of the vendors be required to accept these standards. This arrangement could benefit patients enormously in terms of quality of care, increases in safety, and a big reduction in expenses.

A fourth approach is to provide easily accessible information on drug pricing, along with comparisons of brand-name and generic drugs and of brand-name and generic or OTC substitute drugs with equal efficacy. Physicians need easy access to this type of information so that they will know, for example, that a prescription for the anti-inflammatory betamethasone cream costs $68 compared to the OTC hydrocortisone cream for less than $2.00. Or that the Prevpac costs $350, but would only cost about $150 if they prescribed the less expensive Prilosec proton pump inhibitor instead of the higher-priced Prevacid. Physicians want to know this information but cannot access it readily. As a result, they do what most of us would do and fall back on what they have heard or read most recently, rather than taking away from their short time with a patient to find out the current specifics.

Misconception: *Comparative effectiveness research is nothing but a government method to begin care rationing.*

EVIDENCE-BASED CARE

Another approach to reducing the costs of care is to maximize evidence-based care. A great deal of work still needs to be done to educate physicians on evidence-based use of procedures, drugs, and devices. For example, efforts across the country focus on hospitals to ensure that a patient admitted with pneumonia or a heart attack gets certain basic, well-understood, and proven approaches. For pneumonia, this effort might include checking the patient's oxygen saturation level, getting the antibiotics started shortly after admission to the hospital, and, where appropriate, teaching the patient about smoking cessation before leaving the hospital. The truth is that there is plenty of evidence-based, i.e., well-substantiated, information we physicians should know about but simply do not. Usually these guidelines are straightforward, given the sorts of circumstances I've mentioned.

It still is important, however, to allow a physician to decide what is in the best interest of an individual patient. The insurance company should not make that decision. If the physician wishes to treat a patient in a manner that differs from the norm, then he or she should be allowed to do so, and the insurance should pay the tab. The physician needs to be clear with the patient that the suggested approach is not the standard one and then explain why the physician feels that in this particular situation a different approach may be more appropriate. All of this information also needs to be spelled out clearly in the patient's record. In short, decisions regarding a patient's medical care should be the physician's prerogative but with the understanding *and* consent of the patient. Now here's a caveat about insurance on this issue. When a person buys insurance, it is perfectly reasonable for that person to choose an insurance policy that only covers standard care or evidence-based care. Without extra options, the policy will probably be less expensive, but the person buying the policy should understand the implications of his or her choice up front. It is better to have an affordable policy that covers all appropriate evidence-based medicine than not carrying one because a policy with supplemental features is unaffordable. But there is obviously a trade-off. The important issue is for everyone to understand the rules clearly before an issue develops.

As I have mentioned previously, a major problem is that the consumer is most often left out of the decision when purchasing the insurance, as government policy has shifted it to the employer. In addition, policy language and rules are virtually impossible to understand and interpret, even by the insurer's own staff!

Evidence-based medicine to some degree is a new concept, but in truth it goes back to the beginnings of medicine. The idea is that a physician will offer care that is supported by tested scientific evidence, such as a well-done clinical trial that compares treatment approach A to approach B. It might mean comparing a new drug to an older, established drug or a new technology such as the virtual colonoscopy via CT scan to the standard approach using a colonoscope. Once the data is in, we need to proceed based on that evidence. Medicare, for instance, ruled in 2009 that because the virtual colonoscopy has not been proven to be as good as the visual colonoscopy, as least to Medicare's satisfaction, it will not pay for it. Many are challenging Medicare's decision, but it did not ban virtual colonoscopies. You can choose to have one done if, in consultation with your physician, it still seems to be the best for you; but you will be required to pay for it yourself. Meanwhile, Medicare accepts that the expensive procedures of immediate angioplasty and the insertion of a stent will improve the survival and quality of life for those who have had a heart attack. So Medicare covers these procedures.

The stimulus bill passed in February 2009, the American Recovery and Reinvestment Act of 2009, includes $1.1 billion to begin comparative effectiveness reviews over a two-year period. Within nineteen weeks of passage, an arm of the National Academy of Sciences, the Institute of Medicine (IOM), in its report *Initial National Priorities for Comparative Effectiveness Research* recommended a hundred proposed specific areas for initial investigation. The IOM recommendations put substantial emphasis on evaluating the effectiveness of the health-care *delivery* system, including elements of safety and quality, instead of conducting evaluations that would be comparing, say, drug A to drug B. The institute explained its heavy emphasis this way: "Research topics categorized in this group focus on comparing how or where services are provided, rather than which services are provided. . . . An early investment in comparative effectiveness research (CER) should focus on learning how to make services more effective."[1]

A case in point relates to the treatment of heart attacks. It has been well proven that getting the patient's blocked artery(ies) opened with angioplasty within ninety minutes is highly beneficial in both the short term and the long term. But only a minority of patients actually has the procedure done at all or in the prescribed time frame. So the IOM is encouraging an evaluation of the process, not the procedure, and why it does not function adequately for many patients.

There are those who vociferously argue that that this type of research is nothing but a method to ration care, akin to the British National Institute for Health and Clinical Excellence (NICE) system, which decides if a drug or device will be paid for in the national health-care system. CER is essentially different, as the legislation specifically states that the data cannot be used to determine insurance coverage decisions. Costs, however, will be addressed in the CER process. For example, a new drug or technology may be effective but is still no more effective than other less expensive drugs or devices. This data will be invaluable to the physician and the patient who, together, can then make an informed decision. In the end, high-quality information from these evaluations will understandably threaten the manufacturers (drug, device, and testing companies) and purveyors (hospitals and physicians) of technologies that are equally effective but much more expensive. Affected businesses will fight back.

Another concern is that the results of evaluations will represent the "average" patient's response, but an individual patient might well respond differently; that is, he or she might benefit from a drug that does not have value for others. Here again, the data might help inform the physician when, and under what circumstances, a particular course of action might be most advantageous or most disadvantageous. Three patients with prostate cancer, for instance, could and probably should have much different treatment. The fifty-year-old man with an apparently more aggressive tumor, after learning the various options, might select a radical prostectomy in hopes of a cure. He might choose to go to a surgeon or center that routinely and frequently uses the new robotic approach because, in the right hands, it can improve effectiveness but result in fewer negative side effects. This decision is an expensive but probably appropriate choice. The sixty-five-year-old man with a less aggressive tumor might choose to be treated with radioactive seeds, and an eighty-year-old might select watchful waiting. The point is that in this case, the physician and the patient need good, solid information when considering options and then to reach a decision that is most appropriate for that patient given his tumor, age, family setting, and other personal considerations.

The opportunity to substitute more cost-effective strategies over those that are less so will mean equal or better outcomes at a lower cost. As discussed in various examples throughout this book, in medicine today significant costs could be saved by using a less expensive drug, device, test, or procedure, or, indeed, none at all. Sound research will assist in making the decision clear.

The most difficult choices come when deciding whether to use a new technology (drug, test, device, and so on) that is perhaps somewhat more effective than that currently available but is exceptionally expensive. An example here might be one of the new anticancer drugs that offers patients a few extra months of survival but at a cost of more than $50,000.

The goal is to encourage physicians to shift from using less effective to more effective approaches and concurrently to advise physicians on the cost implications of their decisions. Getting the patient involved in the decision making and providing high-quality, clearly presented information will undoubtedly both improve quality and reduce costs. There should be little excuse for any physician to be an inefficient provider when cost-effective approaches are both known and available.

The issue of new technologies is clearly quite important in the continuing rise of health-care costs. They need to be addressed using some of the approaches I have outlined. What we do not need are various rationing attempts, but they will undoubtedly come if physicians do not find more productive and cost-effective approaches to using new technologies appropriately.

Misconception: *We need to have many systems in place to detect fraud and abuse. Without them, costs would skyrocket even further.*

FRAUD AND ABUSE

The true extent of health-care insurance payment fraud is unknown, but private insurers estimate it is at least $60 billion (or 3 percent of total annual spending.)

The federal government's estimates are higher, or at least $72 billion in costs to the U.S. Treasury.

The U.S. government reported in early 2011 that it had recaptured about $4 billion in 2010 from cases of fraud. It convicted in 2010 slightly more than seven hundred defendants, or a hundred more than in 2009. Some of these cases were for relatively small amounts, but others were for substantial sums of money. Many in Congress believe that the government should push even harder. While no one should believe that confronting fraud and abuse will produce a substantial reduction in the overall costs of American medical care, fraud is egregious and should be actively pursued.

Fraud is submitting a bill for a service never provided, for instance, "up-coding" a visit or hospitalization to a level beyond that provided, or "unbundling" the code rather than submitting the service with the "bundled" code. Most often it is done out of negligence, meaning that the billing clerk in the doctor's office or hospital did not fully understand the rules. However, it is still fraud to bill for treatment that was not performed. In another instance, the specialist physician who says that he is only called upon to see the "sickest of the sick" in the hospital bills all of his cases at the highest category (level 5), no matter what he actually does with the patient. It is fraud, though, if he does not document in the chart that he in fact had provided level-5 services to a patient. A second example is a specialist physician who states he does a certain set of activities for all patients with the same condition. It is abuse and probably fraud if he does a test or procedure (for example, a urologist who does an ultrasound procedure on every patient looking for residual urine after voiding) that a specific patient does not require.

In both of these examples there are no consumer-driven control mechanisms. If I go to the tailor to have a button sewn on my coat and he charges me $5.00, I may think that amount is a fair price. If I see a physician for fifteen minutes and he bills me $50, I may think that is fair as well. If he bills me $300, though, I might think that charge is outrageous. But he does not bill me. His bill goes to the insurer, or third-party payer (TTP), who accepts or rejects the claim. When I receive a statement from the TTP, I find it confusing at best, so I look at what I owe as a deductible or co-pay. If that amount seems reasonable, I ignore the rest. Basically, our payment system eliminates me as an incentivized monitor of the charge for the service that I had.

Then there are the gross examples of fraud. Imagine a podiatrist who obtains a contract to clip toenails for the residents at a nursing home. He comes in weekly and tends to those who need him but submits bills for all of the residents. This practice is stealing. The nursing home resident probably never sees the Medicare statement, though, and the relative who is responsible will probably ignore it or assume it was for an actual service. Another example is a physician who frequently sees a patient with a chronic illness, probably an older person, and submits claims for extra visits that never occurred. This physician is committing outright fraud, but the patient may never realize that he or she and the government have been bilked. Usually these types of criminals only get caught when an alert claims processor or a scanning program recognizes the provider probably could not have seen that many patients.

What can be done? Fraud and abuse need to be minimized, but a major part of the problem is our unnecessarily complex payment system. So we need a simplified system for claim submissions and a more straightforward claim methodology; reducing the level of visit classifications would also help. We need better accountability systems, and the electronic medical record might be of assistance here. Further, the patient must have a functional role in increasing accountability. Having a high-deductible policy will give the patient an incentive to review the bill and ensure it is appropriate for the services rendered. Having the patient sign off at the end of a visit that he or she actually received the care to be billed would be useful as well.

Cutting back on fraud and abuse needs to be done. Unfortunately, wherever there is a huge amount of money at stake—and health care is a multitrillion-dollar industry—some people will try to take advantage, including organized crime. But we also need to remember that there is a huge amount of waste. Curbs on fraud will probably not do much to curtail waste and, indeed, merely may add further restrictions and mandates that add time and costs without improving patient care. It is a delicate balance.

10

The High Cost of Poor Safety and Low-Quality Care

Misconception: *Safety is a problem of poor care but is not a significant cost issue.*

Angela Stepnick, a fifty-three-year-old widow, had a number of medical problems but took only two medications—a thyroid replacement and an antianxiety drug called Xanax (alprazolam). One day she called and said she felt terrible. I told her to come right over. She was obviously seriously dehydrated, yet she said she was thirsty and drinking lots of fluids. She was hospitalized, kept on her two medications, given intravenous fluids, and given some tests to figure out the cause of the problem. Everything came back negative, and she felt fine within twenty-four hours. She went home, but I felt uncomfortable since we had no explanation for her problem.

The next day she called back, "It is starting up all over again." When I asked if she had any idea what was occurring, she replied, "Well, remember I picked up a new refill for the Xanax a week ago. The label said alprazolam generic, but the pills looked different from the last time. I figured it was just a new company making it. But it looks a lot like the 'water pill' you had me take a few years ago after my heart attack." I told her to come right in and bring the pills with her. They were a diuretic, Lasix (furosemide), and not alprazolam despite the label on the pharmacy's vial. Clearly the pharmacist had made a mistake, and my patient had paid the price of a hospitalization and feeling very poorly because the furosemide did what it is supposed to do, that is, made her urinate out salt and water. And the cost to the system was more than $5,000 for the hospitalization and the testing.

PATIENT SAFETY: A CRITICAL COMPONENT OF IMPROVED QUALITY AND REDUCED COSTS

I wrote extensively about preventable medical errors in *The Future of Medicine*, so I will be brief here. We know that about 100,000 deaths per year in the United States result from preventable medical errors. This total is about three times the number of deaths due to car accidents, five times the number of homicides, and sixteen times the number of U.S. servicemen and women killed in Iraq and Afghanistan since the start of hostilities in 2003. Perhaps 100,000 is higher than the actual statistic, but more likely the number is too low. Of course, patients also suffer many nonfatal errors that cause some level of harm, discomfort, or inconvenience. Add to these totals the number of hospital-acquired infections and their resultant deaths, and the numbers become mind-boggling. So here I will focus on some of the most prevalent problems, their costs, and how they can be prevented.

I need to begin by saying that physicians (along with other providers, including hospitals) need to take a much more active and aggressive role in reducing errors and hospital-acquired infections. A hospital-acquired infection is essentially what the term says—an infection that developed while the individual was in the hospital. As with preventable errors, there are about 100,000 deaths per year due to these infections, which often stem from errors as well or from providers paying less-than-adequate attention to care parameters, and they cost in excess of $6 billion to $7 billion per year! Today's hospital is packed with older, sicker individuals who are more susceptible to infection. Many are debilitated, have diseases, or are receiving treatments that render them more prone to developing an infection. They need to be protected from infection.

A common procedure used with many sick individuals is to insert a central venous catheter—that is, an intravenous line into a vein—and thread it up toward the heart, where the vein is much larger. It is then used for administering fluids or drugs, drawing blood, or measuring internal pressures in the body. Many lines get infected (about 80,000 per year), and the patients' resulting infections lead to many additional days in the hospital and an added cost burden of about $40,000 each. Further, 30–40 percent of these patients die. It does not need to be so. A fairly simple checklist approach, if scrupulously followed, will prevent the vast majority of infections. The steps include having only a fully qualified and certified physician place the catheter; ensuring that he or she first washes his or her hands and uses full, sterile precautions, as done in the operating room, including wearing a gown, mask, and gloves; using a neck vein and not a groin vein for insertion; using a Clorhexidine scrub of the site; carefully placing a sterile dressing moistened with Clorhexidine on the insertion site when finished, and removing the catheter as soon as it is no longer absolutely essential. These steps are not impossible or even difficult to follow. It is important that they are followed every time and without exception. It will mean fewer deaths, less time in the hospital for the patient, and a major cost savings.

One of the keys to success in improving the quality of care is that providers should always use a checklist of what needs to be done for any procedure. Not only does it serve as a good reminder of the steps to be followed, but it also enhances teamwork. Since a physician and a nurse insert the catheter together, the checklist works for both of them. An important principle is that the nurse has the power to stop the procedure if the physician does not follow the checklist. This situation is analogous to the copilot in the cockpit who has the authority to delay the takeoff if the captain does not complete each of the proscribed steps. Critical to success is training both the doctor and the nurse to ensure that the nurse not only has the authority but also feels empowered to use that authority if need be.

Infections at the site of surgery are also far too common. As with catheter-related infections, they can be largely prevented. The steps, similar to those outlined for catheterization, are straightforward and have proven the test of time. Again, the key is to have a checklist and to follow it exactly, every time.

You are probably aware that many bacteria have become resistant to commonly used antibiotics. We often read about MRSA, the acronym for methicillin-resistant *Staphylococcus aureus*, but there are many others such as multiple drug-resistant *Pseudomonas* or *Acinetobacter*. One reason for their frequency is that antibiotics are overused in the hospital, including those few antibiotics that are still effective for these germs. Another dangerous problem related to the overuse of antibiotics is *Clostridium difficile*–associated diarrhea, which is caused by a toxin from the bacteria. Hospitals need an antibiotic stewardship program that both limits the use of certain antibiotics and ensures that an expert, either an infectious disease specialist or a pharmacist well trained in antibiotic management, reviews each patient's situation within twenty-four hours of when an antibiotic is ordered by the patients' physician. Stewardship programs have proven valuable for patient care and have saved medium-sized hospitals about $1 million or more per year.

It so happens that many patients arrive at the hospital already colonized— that is medical speak for carrying the germs on the skin, in the mouth, or in the intestines—with a resistant bacteria. The hospital will have swabs of these areas obtained at admission and sent to the laboratory. Since it takes about forty-eight hours for most hospital microbiology laboratories to detect and identify the resistant bacteria (there are some exceptions with new rapid detection and identification systems), it follows that every patient should be in a single room. Indeed, there are some facility design parameters that are important and valuable for reducing hospital-acquired infections. First on the list is to have every patient in a single room with a private toilet. Sinks need to be located near the door to the room as must a wall dispenser with an alcohol-based hand disinfectant. No one should be allowed to enter the room without using one or the other. The air should be filtered with a high-efficiency particulate system, and there should be multiple air exchanges per hour. The water system must be properly designed so that bacteria cannot contaminate it. The room needs to be designed so that it can be readily cleaned. Sometimes this may mean use of newer techniques, such as hydrogen peroxide vaporization, which is admittedly very expensive, rather than routine scrubbing with a disinfectant.

It is also important to reduce the number of times a patient is transferred. Transfers lead to more hospital-acquired infections for the patient. Moving a patient from one location to another also means a transfer to a new nursing staff and is inherently fraught with critical information loss. For the staff, transfers involve more paperwork, rather than bedside care, and it is when more injuries, such as back strains, occur. Single bedrooms, especially those designed for varying levels of patient acuity (that is, how sick the patient is), lead to reduced transfers, fewer errors, and lower costs. Despite the benefits of not moving the patient, though, there are often good reasons to do so, such as getting maximum utilization of critical staff members.

There is good data showing that the lighting in hospitals is usually inadequate. Once we are older than age forty, we need more light to see well. The average age of the nursing staff in most hospitals is older than forty-five years; so extra light is important. It is also important in the pharmacy; improved lighting when medications are prepared reduces errors.

Finally a major problem in hospitals (and in nursing homes) is patient falls. These accidents cause more injuries even though they are less common than medication errors. Most falls occur when the patient needs to go to the bathroom, as evidenced by urine on the floor where the patient fell. Since patients are older, sicker, and on many medications (often more than ten), they may be drowsy or confused and try to crawl out of bed despite the bed's guardrails being used. In fact, bed rails are a real problem; they do not work. The patient simply climbs over them and then falls even farther. The steps to prevent falls are to encourage voiding before sleeping, to avoid drugs that confuse, to have a readily available nurse buzzer, to keep care articles within reach, to eliminate electrical cords and clutter, to install hand rails along the wall to the bathroom, to have a short walk to the toilet and a wide bathroom door, and, perhaps most important, to encourage family members to be present.

This compendium of trouble spots in the hospital is not comprehensive, but if providers will use a checklist when inserting central lines, create a program of antibiotic stewardship, pay attention to preventing patient falls, use properly designed single rooms, encourage fewer patients transfers, improve task lighting, and rigorously enforce hand hygiene, then hospital-acquired infections and patient falls, along with costs, will decline dramatically. It will result in much better patient care and a reduction in unnecessary expenses and preventable medical errors.

BROKEN MALPRACTICE SYSTEM

Closely related to the patient safety issue is our broken malpractice system. Frankly, it is a disaster of a system that does not improve care and costs too much. Physicians paid about $6.3 billion per year in insurance in 2002 (and rates have increased markedly since then), costs that are ultimately reflected in the patient's bill for care. The process of dealing with malpractice claims is slow, secrecy abounds, and communication is always poor. The patient's lawyer gets about 33–40 percent of any payment, meaning the patient only receives about 60–67 percent. This system encourages secrecy, discourages apology, and does not prevent similar errors in the future. This system is exactly the opposite of what we need.

Let's start with the basics. If a patient is harmed, it is essential—indeed, a moral and ethical obligation—that the physician explains what went wrong to the patient in straightforward, simple, and understandable terms. This explanation should be followed with an immediate apology, one that is heartfelt and straightforward without casting blame on anyone else. Then the patient should be compensated promptly. But with today's system, physicians are often encouraged not to apologize for any errors, because an apology might be interpreted as an admission of guilt and could be used against them in court. Further, the entire system is set up to slow down the timely compensation of the patient. If it could be corrected, then it would also be possible to discuss errors openly with other staff members, to do a root cause analysis of why the error occurred, and then to fix or improve systems to prevent a similar error from occurring to another patient in the future. This process would be better for the injured patient, better for the doctor or nurse who made the error, and better for everyone else because it would help reduce similar errors going forward.

Rather than the current tort system, the better approach would be using a nonjudicial mediation process that ensures prompt and adequate payment for harm. The focus should be on rapid resolution, not blame, and the payment should be for economic damages with a cap on payments for noneconomic damages, or for pain and suffering. Using the same guidelines, there also could be special courts to render judgments. As with special courts for tax issues and for complicated trade issues, a judge or other appropriate judicial officer could hear and settle malpractice cases. Outcomes could be linked to licensing boards to ensure that providers are required to attend remediation training or education when found to be deficient. The costs of either of these approaches would be much less than today's system, and the patient who is harmed would garner a much larger share of any settlement.

It is important to state that these proposed changes will not absolve the individual who makes the mistake of responsibility and accountability. Rather, they will create an environment and a system whereby errors are discussed openly and reviewed carefully and whereby new approaches are put into place to prevent the same errors from reoccurring.

"To err is human," so it follows that we will all make mistakes. The key is to have systems in place that will help prevent an individual from making a mistake, or once the mistake is made, the system will catch it and remediate before harm can occur to the patient. Here is an example. Sometimes a hospital patient's blood potassium level drops dangerously low, so physicians give an intravenous injection of potassium in the form of potassium chloride. But if the patient gets too much potassium chloride, or gets too much too quickly, the level of potassium in the blood can rise dangerously high and, in turn, can have an adverse effect on the heart, even causing it to stop beating. For years, potassium chloride has come packaged in vials with one of two concentrations, low and high. Although the concentration is noted clearly on the vial's label, it is possible to pick up the vial of the higher concentration, mistake it for the lower concentration, and then give too much to the patient. The individual who made the mistake undoubtedly and unquestionably caused harm, and it can be a serious error with the patient's life at stake. Fortunately, over time, reports of these errors from hospitals all across the country had been sent into the Joint Commission on Accreditation of Healthcare Organizations, and officials there recognized that they were seeing a fair number of such reports. They studied the situation carefully and then made the recommendation that the high-concentration vial simply should not be available on patient care units where this type of mistake can be made. As a result, a rare event in any one hospital, but one that was occurring nevertheless in hospitals everywhere, has been largely prevented across the country.

This type of approach needs to be followed all the time, with in-hospital reviews of errors both to see if there is a common pattern and to develop a methodology to prevent the error from reoccurring. My recommendation, thus, will result in a better system for the injured patient with a prompt explanation, an apology, and compensation while at the same time encouraging the collection of the data that can be used to decrease errors in the future.

What about accountability? Would "bad apples" get off scot-free? Accountability in this system remains absolutely essential; again, it is all about balancing rights with responsibilities. Consider the physician who knows full well the importance of hand washing to prevent hospital-acquired infections yet fails to wash regularly. Assuming that sinks and soap are available, after an initial warning, a repeat offense demands accountability. Perhaps a penalty, such as a two-week exclusion from the operating room or from admitting to the hospital, both of which put a serious crimp in his or her income, would suffice. Hospital executives to date have been loath to enforce such rules because the physician in question might take his or her patients elsewhere. But the hospital's board of trustees and the CEO must insist that basic standards of practice will be honored, period.

Accountability and error mitigation are both essential. We know that more than 100,000 people per year die and even more are injured because of preventable medical errors. Despite the landmark publication a decade ago by the Institute of Medicine, which resulted in much intense discussion and even substantial action by hospital boards and staff across the country, preventable errors are still a huge problem. Doctors (and hospitals) are quick to say that the current tort system of malpractice is unfair and burdens them with very expensive insurance. It does. Yet doctors and hospitals have not done enough to control the problem of medical errors. Until they do, it is unfair to expect legislatures to grant much relief.

To reiterate, it would be wise to overhaul the malpractice system and create one that encourages error explanations, apologies, and prompt compensation along with careful analyses and follow-up actions to help prevent similar errors in the future and concurrently to hold physicians, nurses, and other professionals accountable for their actions with meaningful sanctions.

11

The Costs of Too Much Care

Misconception: *As with other elements of the marketplace, giving patients more control of their health-care expenditures will lead to lower costs.*

I went to my internist and showed him a rash on my calf. He diagnosed dermatitis and recommended that I use a steroid cream to eradicate it. When he gave me a prescription for betamethasone, I asked him why he did not suggest simply using hydrocortisone. His response seemed logical: The betamethasone is stronger and would resolve the problem quickly. I went to the pharmacy, and while the pharmacist was preparing my prescription, I noticed that hydrocortisone was available over the counter then for $1.98. When my prescription for betamethasone was ready, I was presented with a bill for $69. When I protested, I was told that if I had not had a drug discount card, the betamethasone tube would have cost $83. If I had been really smart, I would have declined the betamethasone, purchased the hydrocortisone, and accepted the fact that it would take a few more days to resolve my rash. Instead, like most people, I paid the money and went on my way. By the way, since I had a high-deductible insurance policy, I paid the entire amount for that tube of steroid cream. So was I stupid, or a rather typical patient who thought that since my doctor had prescribed the medicine, I should go with his advice? OK, so I was probably stupid, but as with most of you in similar circumstances, I heeded my doctor's advice. When I talked to my physician later, he had no idea that betamethasone cost that much more than hydrocortisone and was frankly surprised. This episode has stuck in my mind over the past few years and, as I hope to demonstrate, was the first step in my education and ultimate change in perspective about how patients can help control costs.

I had always thought that patients' decisions about medical expenditures were quite different from those we make about other major expenditures, such as buying a new dishwasher or a new car. In those cases we comparison shop, check out reviews and research, and are not afraid to ask many questions. Often, we do not do the same with medical expenditure recommendations from our physician.

DRUG COSTS: UNITED STATES VERSUS OTHER COUNTRIES

We often hear that drugs in the United States cost more than they do in other countries and that if only we could re-import them from Canada, for example, we could save a substantial amount of money. The individual with a complex, chronic illness usually takes multiple medications that are on patent and hence reasonably expensive, and he or she finds that insurance does not cover all the costs. No wonder these individuals and our politicians both feel that it should be appropriate to re-import exactly the same drugs at a much lower price from another country. But let's consider that a large proportion of pharmaceutical research is done in the United States, and the drug companies need to recoup their research and development (R&D) expenses. Currently these outlays can run almost a billion dollars per drug by the time it is approved by the Food and Drug Administration. It takes many years from the time a new compound is first discovered in the basic research laboratories until it has completed all of the laboratory tests, the animal toxicity testing, and finally the human testing before the FDA can approve it on the basis of both its efficacy and its safety. So the price of a new drug when it comes on the market includes these R&D costs, and they are one of the reasons why a new drug is so expensive. Many countries, however, impose price controls and, in effect, limit what a company can sell the drug for, let's say $6 rather than $10, which is what it costs in the United States. Because $6 is still above the drug's marginal cost, or the actual cost to manufacture it, the drug company agrees to sell the medication in that country at the $6 price. This arrangement means that America is funding the research and development of the new drug and other countries are not. It is also why a drug might cost less in Canada than it does directly across the border in a northern U.S. state.

What can we do about the high cost of drugs in the United States as compared to other countries? The problem with re-importation from, say, Canada is that the Food and Drug Administration would have to make great efforts to verify that the drug being purchased from another country is indeed the drug that was manufactured by the company in question. At some point, when medications have their packages individually marked with a radio frequency identification (RFID) tags, which would allow companies to track the drugs when they leave the manufacturer, or even if individual pills and capsules have some form of identification, then it might be possible to safely re-import drugs. Until that time, I would make a different suggestion. The federal government purchases about half of all drugs and devices sold in the United States through Medicare, Medicaid, the Department of Defense, and the Department of Veterans Affairs. The federal government should mandate that it will not purchase a drug or device that is sold in another country at a lower price than it is sold for in the United States. If a company wants to sell its product for a lower price in another country, so be it, but it will have to sell it at that same price in the United States. This will force a reduction in prices for American purchasers and spread the R&D costs equally across all purchasers. An exception should be made for selling drugs and devices in underdeveloped countries. Many manufacturers are willing to sell their products there at a marked discount since it is well understood that these countries' populations simply cannot afford to pay the market prices.

DOCTORS' PRESCRIBING PATTERNS

Another problem with drugs is that many doctors write a prescription instead of recommending a lifestyle change that could eliminate the need for a drug. In chapter 9 is an example of using drugs for reflux esophagitis, or heartburn, rather than suggesting that the patient change his or her lifestyle to eat a smaller meal in the evening, to add a few hours between dinner and bedtime to aid digestion, to raise the head of the bed, and to drink less alcohol and caffeine. The trouble is that it takes time to talk to a patient about such lifestyle changes, and unfortunately that extra time is not reimbursed by insurance.

Another problem is that doctors often prescribe a brand-name drug instead of a generic drug. In the example of heartburn, doctors prescribe the branded Nexium, which is still under patent, instead of prescribing or recommending the now OTC drug Prilosec. And the choice between betamethasone or hydrocortisone at the start of this chapter is another example. Part of the problem is that physicians often are not fully cognizant of the difference in costs from drug to drug.

Physicians are also regaled regularly with sales pitches from drug company representatives. Over the years I found most of the representatives to be honest and hardworking. But their job is still to convince physicians that the drug from their drug company is superior to the one from another company. Often the difference between drugs can be real but relatively minor, such as the differences between Prilosec, Nexium, and Prevacid. That said, the drug company representative responsible for Prevacid will point out its supposed advantages compared to the others and certainly will make the case that the Prevpac to treat the *H. pylori* cause of stomach ulcers makes life a lot easier for patients, ensuring that the patient will take the three-drug regimen on time and on schedule for the entire fourteen days. It's not a bad sales pitch, except when one examines the big difference in price.

So we must consider at least three issues to understand why drugs run up the costs of health care so much. First, doctors prescribe drugs instead of asking patients to make lifestyle changes. Next, doctors prescribe an ostensibly better drug that is really not that much better but costs a great deal more. And a drug is prescribed that really is not better, but it appears to have an advantage some of the time. All of these matters are exacerbated by the pharmaceutical industry when it advertises directly to the consumer, leading patients to ask their doctors for a prescription for their ailments, such as for restless leg syndrome, and when it encourages doctors to prescribe specific brands of medication without regard to their true necessity or cost. In sum, many expensive, branded drugs are being sold when either no drug is necessary or when a much less expensive drug or a generic equivalent could do the job just as well.

NOT ACCEPTING DEATH AS INEVITABLE

We all know that death is inevitable, but our culture refuses to acknowledge it. Similar to the country-and-western singer who croons, "We all want to go to heaven but not today," we would like to postpone that date with our destiny. For each of us, today is not the day we wish to die; rather, we hope it will be many years in the future. Medicine, of course, is all about denying death, but sometimes death is inevitable and should be allowed to occur without attempts to deny it.

Many physicians see death as a failure, but it is not necessarily a failure. It is simply the certain outcome of life. But frequently and, indeed, all too often, physicians will recommend another course of therapy, and patients will ask their physicians if there isn't "one last thing" that could be tried. These efforts stem from normal human reactions and emotions, and sometimes another approach exists that can be not only useful but also effective. But when there is no recourse, it is important for the physician, in particular, and for the patient and the patient's family to understand that there is a limit to what medical science can do. At this point, the physician, the patient, and the patient's family need to have a realistic conversation about the situation and decide how to proceed appropriately. This issue has nothing to do with "death panels" or the rationing of care. Instead, it is about ensuring everyone understands all of the options and their implications for care.

The important point I want to make here is that when no additional therapy can be effective, it is appropriate to allow for death with dignity and comfort in an appropriate setting. To attempt to deny death means a major consumption of scarce medical resources such as hospitalizations, aggressive but ineffective drug therapies, days or weeks in the intensive care unit, multiple imaging tests, and laboratory evaluations. All of these efforts are usually for naught yet bring added discomfort, pain, and anxiety. It is an enormous misuse of resources with little or no benefit.

I am reminded of an example from when I had recently begun my residency after a year of internship at Yale New Haven Hospital. An elderly gentleman was admitted to the ICU with a major pulmonary embolus, or a blood clot that had moved up from his leg and was seriously affecting his breathing and heart function. The intern and I, along with his personal physician, worked hard to save his life. But although he survived the first few days, it became clear that he would be dependent on a respirator, and he remained comatose. We continued to care for him, but he died a few weeks later of pneumonia, essentially unchanged. All of our efforts had been in vain and had probably bankrupted his now widow, no matter how good her insurance might have been.

Here is another, more recent personal story about end-of-life care. I had taken care of a lovely woman for more than thirty years, first for her cancer, which fortunately had been cured, and then for a series of other medical problems, including a significant endocrine problem, a heart attack that required open-heart surgery, and a level of anxiety and depression after her husband died. She obtained her flu vaccine annually, but that winter developed a pneumonia caused by a virus called parainfluenza. Her adult son brought her to the emergency room, and she was admitted. Over the next two days her condition substantially worsened and she was moved to the ICU, where a breathing machine was used to assist her. I honestly thought that if we could get through a few more days, the infection would probably start to clear and she could go back home again. I also knew that her situation was precarious and that in all likelihood we would need to insert a tube into her airway and place her on a respirator. I also knew this procedure was not something she would want to do.

About that time her son, who was in his mid-forties, told me that he was feeling quite guilty. "Why?" I asked. He told me that when his mother first became ill a few days before, she had said to him that it was time for her to die and that she really did not want to go to the hospital. He had insisted and brought her in. Now he saw that life for her in the ICU was very difficult, and he wondered if he had made the right decision. He asked if I would please talk to his mother.

So I went into the intensive care unit and turned off all the monitors that were beeping. My patient and I had a good discussion in which I told her that her son loved her deeply and wanted her to survive, but he also did not want to go against her wishes. On his behalf, I told the patient that if she wanted to dispense with the breathing assistance that it was OK. She should feel free to make her own decisions, I advised, and not worry about disappointing either her son or me. I suggested she think about it and not respond right away.

Later in the day, she indicated that she wanted to have everything turned off, knowing full well what that instruction implied. She died peacefully later that evening with her son at her side.

PALLIATIVE CARE

During the health-care reform debate, people made unfortunate references to death panels. No such board was ever in the proposals, but that important part of medical care subsequently was set aside as too toxic to discuss. But end-of-life counseling is quite crucial, as the preceding section suggests. It is good to have such realistic discussions at the beginning of a serious illness; indeed, it is only fair to the patient and the patient's family.

While I don't like the term "palliative care"—it seems to imply only end-of-life care, so I prefer "supportive care"—it is designed to achieve the best possible quality of care and the least suffering possible for the patient. This care is not limited to pain management; it also applies to psychosocial support, spiritual needs, the treatment of any symptoms, and assistance or at least support in decision making. It might involve a complicated pain management program or a simple cup of tea in the afternoon to talk over important issues. Ideally it uses a team approach, including physicians, nurses, social workers, psychologists, chaplains, and others all working together. Palliative care teams have demonstrated their value in improving patients' circumstances and, interestingly, substantially reducing medical care costs.

My experience, and others report the same, is that many physicians are uncomfortable with proposing palliative care. Perhaps it gets at the deep inner concern that they do not want to be seen as giving up on the patient, and perhaps it even forces them to admit that they cannot always cure every patient. Whatever the cause, it is unfortunate because many people who could benefit from early referral to the palliative care team are not getting that assistance. Most large hospitals now have such teams; it behooves the patient or family to ask about them.

PERFORMING UNNECESSARY TESTS AND PROCEDURES

Most physicians do not want to admit it, and perhaps do not even recognize it, but the truth is that physicians often perform unnecessary tests and procedures. Because a procedure or test is available and fits the patient's circumstances, it does not necessarily need to be done. But many physicians' motto seems to be "We do what we know how to do or can do." Some think physicians order tests or procedures because of malpractice concerns. "If I don't do that test and then it turns out that the patient had such-and-such, I may be at malpractice risk!" It might be part of the problem, but it is also because physicians are trained to run down every possibility. Every physician also knows the old adage, "When you hear hoof beats, think of horses, not zebras." The problem is that we seem to worry about zebras, meaning uncommon or even rare diseases, to an excessive extent, and physicians order procedures, laboratory tests, and referrals to another specialist for a second opinion when none of it is really necessary.

One major problem is that physicians are not compensated adequately for taking careful histories, so their instinct is to order tests and procedures instead. (Again, if primary care physicians reduce the number of patients they care for to about five hundred, they could give each patient adequate time and attention, but, of course, you or your insurance will pay a larger amount per visit or per year of contracted services for this comprehensive form of primary care. With this model, the quality of care goes up, the use of unwarranted tests and procedures goes down dramatically, and a big reduction in expenditures is realized.) All too frequently, the patient's PCP will send the patient to a specialist for a second opinion as well. This step can be appropriate when necessary, but often it is done because the generalist simply is not willing to take the time to explore the patient's case history carefully. Of course, the specialist feels the need to "do something" when the patient comes in for the consultation and may order a second round of tests or procedures. The second part of the problem is that new tests such as CT scans and MRIs and blood chemical tests are easy to order, can give extensive information in return, and often quickly find the cause of a problem. But they can be overutilized.

At the far end of the spectrum, I was told recently about a physician in a poor area of Africa who does a simple, no-cost test to try and diagnose diabetes. He asks the patient to go in the backyard of his office area and urinate. He waits twenty minutes and looks to see if ants have found the area. If they have, then there is sugar in the urine. He says that he would like to do a regular test for sugar in the urine or better yet a blood test of the levels of glucose in the bloodstream, but he knows that his patients are poor and simply cannot afford it. This system is an extreme of not overusing expensive laboratory tests, but too often physicians go in the opposite direction when it is not truly necessary. But since the insurance pays for the test, the patient does not question the doctor's recommendation.

Here is an example of an overused, expensive procedure. When a patient has persistent reflux esophagitis that does not respond to basic approaches, most gastroenterologists and internists will suggest doing an endoscopy. It involves running a tube about the thickness of your index finger through your mouth, down your throat, down the esophagus, and into the stomach. The gastroenterologist can get a good look at the stomach lining, the lining of the upper small intestines, and the area where the stomach and the esophagus come together. In all likelihood the test will be negative, but the gastroenterologist wants to know if you have an esophageal cancer. While uncommon, and certainly more uncommon in younger adults, it does occur, and the physician is concerned that the persistent symptoms of reflux esophagitis may suggest a cancer. Fair enough, but the test is expensive (usually more than $1,000), makes patients anxious in the interim until it is actually done, has a low but definite risk of complications, and is unlikely to find anything significant. And when the gastroenterologist reports to the patient that everything looks fine, the patient will still have the heartburn.

The physician is paid a reasonable fee for doing the endoscopy, but unfortunately he or she might not take the time to also explore the patient's history, which might reveal, in some patients, that the real problem is the patient's sensitivity to wheat or the gluten in the wheat. In that case, if the patient stops eating foods containing gluten, such as wheat, rye, and barley, the reflux will subside. The endoscopy, though, will not detect wheat sensitivity (unless it is the less common but serious celiac disease). So procedures tend to be overused, especially in a patient who has a chronic problem and repeatedly returns to the physician seeking a resolution. All of these combined tests and procedures add to the cost of American medicine.

PATIENTS CONTROL EXPENDITURES

Having a vested interest in health-care expenditures does make a difference when making health-care decisions, and if the amount of money involved is larger, then it would likely make an even greater difference. I did purchase the much more expensive betamethasone as prescribed, but because my wife and I have a high-deductible Medigap policy, I decided against the special $700 or more repeat look at my vocal cords after my hoarseness improved (see chapter 6). I had asked the speech pathologist if it was really necessary, and she had said, "We always repeat the test because we like to see how the therapy has worked out, but I guess there is no real need for you to do it just now." In effect, she said testing was their preference but not necessary. That comment made my decision easy. This encounter also demonstrates that we need to ask our provider about each test, procedure, and drug and challenge whether it is needed or is the best option in our circumstances.

Similarly, a cardiologist advised me that it was a good idea to get a stress test every year. In discussing this recommendation with my internist, he suggested it was not necessary after obtaining a baseline because I have normal blood pressure, good cholesterol levels, and a normal weight; I exercise regularly; and I don't smoke. He did add that I still could have coronary artery disease and could fall over dead on the way out of his office, but it was quite unlikely. I skipped the repeat stress test.

I used to believe that we buy medical care differently than we do a new dishwasher. We don't have any consumer ratings agency to give us advice. We don't shop three physicians to see whose price is best. Mostly, we follow the advice of our own PCP, provided we are comfortable with him or her. And in general, our physician wants only the best for us, so he or she will refer us to a specialist known to be competent and responsive, will only order tests or procedures that are really needed, will suggest the most appropriate drugs, and in general will look out for our best interests. At least that is the idea.

But we have seen that this model, all too frequently, does not actually work out as well as it should. We need to get more involved on our own behalf. Our incentive should be protecting our own health, but our training is to not question the doctor. If we have to pay for the first $1,000 (or more) of costs out of pocket each year in deductibles, however, we will begin to pay more attention, ask additional questions, debate our options, and insist on transparency, full discussion, and extra information. When we become responsible for our own care, as we should be, the care gets better and the costs come down.

12

We Have Met the Enemy and He Isn't the Insurance Company

Misconception: *The insurance companies are the primary culprits causing insurance premiums to rise.*

Suffering from severe neck pain, Michael Johnson visited a spine surgeon but said up front that he did not want surgery. The surgeon therefore suggested that he visit a pain clinic, where he could get injections to reduce the discomfort. The pain physician injected Novocain into the neck where the nerve roots come out in three places. The idea was that, if effective, the pain would disappear for about six hours. So if it worked, Johnson could return and the physician would repeat the procedure but with another substance that would last about six months. The doctor wanted to be sure that the procedure would be helpful first because the next substance was potentially toxic. The Novocain was not effective, so my friend did not return and is now going to an acupuncturist, whose work seems to be helping. But he was amazed at the price of his recent procedure at the pain clinic: "Over $5,000 for an injection that took less than thirty minutes! I just can't afford that kind of stuff." His bill was for $5,118, but the insurance had disallowed $4,800, paid $234, and left my friend with a co-pay of $84.

You can look at this situation many ways. First, my friend obtained a $5,118 procedure for only $84 out of pocket, which is not bad. You might think, "Gee, if the physician can accept $234 from the insurance company and $84 from the patient as payment in full, then the $4,800 must be bogus at best." Or you might think that it really pays to have insurance because if you did not, then the physician would have expected you to pay the full amount in cash. People who are self-payers really get the raw end of the deal. You need the insurance company to negotiate (or dictate) the best price for you with the provider.

BROKEN INSURANCE SYSTEM

So far we mostly have addressed what the medical profession must do to improve care and reduce costs. But physicians, nurses, pharmacists, and hospitals cannot take on the entire burden. It is absolutely critical to have the insurance carriers be part of the solution.

Today, our system is perverse, with either the government or the employer rather than the patient being the client of the insurer; with the physician essentially working for the insurer rather than for the patient; and the insurers working for the business or the government. This arrangement is atypical of the financial marketplace. The government, both state and federal, sets mandates as to what insurance must cover (for example, cholesterol screening or mammography); moreover, the government, which is the largest single purchaser of insurance, is also the regulator. The patient is a bystander. Since the patient not only pays relatively little to the provider directly, he or she has minimal incentive to be a more knowledgeable and more cost-conscious patient.

We have received good value for the money that the government—largely from the National Institutes of Health through grants to medical school faculty researchers—and the pharmaceutical, biotechnology, and medical device industry has spent on medical research and development. New medicines, for example, have cured many diseases, ameliorated others, and brought relief to millions. Consider, for example, how drugs improve the lives of those with severe depression or cure previously incurable stomach and duodenal ulcers and how angioplasty and stents prevent the progression of heart attacks. We do not get a similarly good value from our various insurance products, however, because in health care all of the usual rational measures of value are missing as a result of misaligned incentives. The physician "works for" the insurer, which, in turn, "works for" the employer or the government. No one works for the patient because the customer and the purchaser of the service are not one and the same.

It will make a major impact if the individual becomes the one who buys the insurance policy. First, it will necessitate a change in tax policy so that the individual is not, as he or she is today, at a disadvantage and buying insurance directly with posttax dollars. And if everyone has a high-deductible policy, they will be incented to watch how their health-care dollars are spent.

COMMERCIAL INSURANCE

The insurance system in this country can best be described as broken. Our insurance system was developed after World War II to cover relatively infrequent but expensive events, such as major procedures and hospitalizations. Indeed, it was often referred to as a "major medical" policy. Now we expect insurance to cover essentially everything from basic care to preventive care to screenings along with catastrophic care. It has become essentially prepaid medical care, but we now have a population with complex, chronic diseases that last a lifetime, diseases the original system was never designed to address.

Our insurance system seems to satisfy essentially no one. One of the biggest frustrations is with the payment system. As a patient you have been frustrated, I am sure, with the multiple forms you have received in the mail, most of which seem complicated, confusing, annoying, and not terribly informative. Let's look at a hypothetical one carefully. You saw your physician for an annual physical examination and the insurance form indicates that the physician entered a bill for $250. That charge is in the third column. The fourth column indicates the amount of money that the insurance company has contracted with the physician for an annual physical exam, or $150. (The physician has accepted this contract because he or she has only two choices—accept or not be part of that insurance company's panel of doctors.) But the next column indicates that the insurance company has reduced it further to $100. The next columns indicate your co-pay percent of 25 percent and then the co-pay amount, leaving in the next column the amount that is eligible for insurance, or $75. If you have a policy with a high deductible, then you are also responsible for the remaining $75. Otherwise, your insurance company will pay your physician $75, and eventually your physician will send you a bill for the $25 co-pay. So after much paperwork, your physician will be paid $100 for an exam that he or she believed was worth $250. You may be satisfied that your insurance company has negotiated the rate down to $100 and that you in turn are only responsible for $25. That fee is not bad for an annual physical exam.

Provider	Service date	Billed charges	Contractual amount	Reduced amount	Eligible for coverage	Co-pay or deductible	Covered	Your share
#12345	01-03-09	$250	$150	$100	$100	25%	$75	$25

Now let's look at the bill from the physician's perspective. He or she needs to pay the rent, the utilities, the office staff, malpractice insurance, other insurance, and himself or herself. Because the insurance company has negotiated a rate of $100 for an annual physical exam, the physician has little choice but to increase the number of patients seen in the course of a day to make ends meet. Because the rent goes up every few years, the utility bills go up every year, and the staff requires regular raises, the only way the physician can hope to maintain even a flat personal salary is to see more patients. The result? When we go to see our physician we are allotted less time. Physicians will say that they are not satisfied with the amount of time they have with each patient, but they feel an obligation to see more patients so that they can cover their expenses.

One of those expenses is to hire billing clerks to interact with the insurance company and to understand all of the intricate policies and rules of the payer. A major problem is that the physician's office often submits bills to the insurance company only to have them rejected. Usually the reason is trivial, but the physician's office staff has to resubmit the claim, adjusting a few simple words or adjusting a procedure code, for example, to make the claim acceptable to the insurance company.

On the other side of the ledger, the insurance company feels that it must go through this sort of process to ensure that it does not end up paying for an inappropriate or unauthorized visit. The insurance company has seen many inappropriate claims or a perfectly appropriate claim that simply isn't covered by the individual patient's insurance. The insurance company will say that false claims and inappropriate claims constitute a fair proportion of the claims submitted and that it must spend an inordinate amount of time and money to have various clerks check and recheck whether each claim is appropriate. I am told that there is about one insurance employee for every two physicians, representing a major waste of money that is not going to patient care.

The hospital situation regarding payments from the insurance carrier is quite similar. The hospital billing office determines who the patient's insurance carrier is and submits a claim after the patient is discharged. As with the physician's office, the hospital's claim is frequently returned, indicating that some part of the form is inadequately completed. Resubmissions required for trivia are commonplace. The hospital must employ large numbers of individuals to bill and verify claims and get them appropriately submitted to the insurance carriers. Frequently the insurance carrier will deny a procedure, a day in the hospital, or a test on the basis that it was not necessary. So hospitals also must hire large numbers of case managers who roam the floors every day to see if a patient should be discharged or if the note in the patient's chart is sufficient to justify that day in the hospital. All of this effort costs money, money that is not going to anyone's direct care. In the end, those costs are borne by whoever is paying the bill whether that is your employer or you or both.

A second set of issues keeping insurance costs high involves mandates. A mandate is the legislative requirement by a state that says the insurance company must cover a particular problem or service. For example, the state might require that any company selling insurance in that state must cover childhood vaccinations, mammography for women older than forty years of age, or acupuncture for lower back pain. Most mandates are valuable, but they add to the cost of insurance. I have advocated for various mandates while I was president in the Maryland Division of the American Cancer Society (ACS). We campaigned for insurance to cover mammography, colonoscopy, and other cancer screening tests on the logical grounds that detecting cancer early, first of all, might save a life. Second, it would reduce costs overall because the cancer would be found early and treated, all at a relatively low expense. But should all these mandates be part of insurance? The sellers of services advocate for mandates in the state legislatures, of course, because they will increase their business. Others see them as a social good, which I did as a member of the ACS. The other advocates of mandates are you and I. Why? Because if it is part of our employer-paid insurance, our out-of-pocket costs go down, and our children's vaccinations and our own mammography or our own colonoscopy are done at little or no cost to us personally. But clearly these mandates raise the cost of insurance.

One of the fundamental problems with commercial insurance is the discrepancy in the tax status between employer-based and individual insurance. Employers who offer health insurance can charge it as an expense of business, thereby reducing their taxes, and the employee's portion of the premium is paid with pretax dollars. An individual who buys the same policy directly will pay for it in posttax, not pretax, dollars. This difference means that the same policy for the same amount of coverage costs a great deal more for the individual who buys his or her own policy directly. I learned this disparity when I retired. My wife and I were not yet sixty-five years old, so we needed to buy our own insurance until Medicare kicked in. Our agent told us that a Blue Cross/Blue Shield policy essentially identical to the policy my wife and I had while I was at work would cost us $13,000, the same amount that my former employer paid Blue Cross/Blue Shield as part of its self-insurance for its employees.

But unless I was self-employed, I could not deduct my health insurance on my federal or state taxes.

Let's also look at insurance from the insurer's perspective. Most policies are not true insurance. Large companies basically self-insure. They use a third-party payer, such as Blue Cross/Blue Shield, Aetna, or UnitedHealthcare, to service their claims. The TTP does an actuarial analysis and tells the company what it will need to pay for the year's coverage, claims, administrative work, and so on. Usually it also includes some true insurance for catastrophic claims, which is especially important for smaller firms that have fewer employees over which to spread the risk. Each state has its own set of mandates, so the mandates of your state are standard in all policies sold by the insurer there. That's the starting point from which your employer can set its own limits and requirements. These stipulations will include how much the employee pays of the cost per person, what the deductible or co-pays will be, and whether certain non-mandated conditions are included for insurance, such as in vitro fertilization or entry into a clinical trial of new drugs or procedures. It is then up to the TPP to interact with the employee, the doctor, the specialist, and the hospital to pay claims and adjudicate disputes. The TPP is in the employ of the business, not the individual employee. Because the TPP is obligated to follow the contract it has with the business, when a physician calls and wants to send the patient for a special procedure, the TPP authorizes it or denies it based on that specific contract. When the patient calls to resolve an issue, it also will be resolved on the basis of the TTP's contract with the business.

It is an interesting system where neither the patient nor the doctor is a client of the insurer's (TPP). This setup certainly runs counter to any other typical business arrangement you might have for professional services.

What needs to be done to improve commercial insurance? Once, not-for-profits such as Blue Cross/Blue Shield provided almost all commercial insurance. I have no personal problem with companies making a profit, but I do think the system would be better if the insurers were nonprofit entities. Particularly important is for state legislatures to eliminate most mandates. There are, of course, a lot of complexities to be resolved, but for simplicity's sake here let everyone have the option to buy a basic Chevy plan, and if an individual wants the equivalent of a Cadillac upgrade, it should be that person's decision to make that choice. One way some have advocated to jump-start this process would be to allow clients to purchase policies across state borders. This move would allow an individual to buy a policy that emanates from a state that does not have so many mandates and, as a result, costs less money. To be sure, less money spent also means less coverage. In effect, this process would institute tiered policies in which the basic level is for everyone, and those who wish to have more coverage would pay an added cost. The basic level might offer similar or even less comprehensive coverage to what basic Medicare provides everyone today who is sixty-five and older. If people want greater coverage, then they could purchase a plan somewhat like the equivalent of today's Medicare wraparound insurance policies, or Medigap. Then, if they want more benefits and are willing to pay a larger sum, a policy that essentially pays for any service, any provider, anywhere could be established. But it is essential that we all have at least a basic level of insurance.

Insurance should be taxed equivalently. The person who buys insurance directly should reap the same tax advantage as the companies that offer it to their employees. Having health insurance untaxed at the corporate level also encourages the creation of excessive insurance programs, or so-called gold-plated policies or Cadillac plans, that are not available to everyone else. These plans are to be taxed under the new reform bill. Originally legislators thought that this measure would only affect the high-level Wall Street types, but many unions had negotiated similar plans, so the tax was deferred until 2018.

Insurance tends to work on the basis of payments for a visit or a procedure. This system encourages excessive visits and procedures since they bring in more dollars to the provider. It discourages what is really needed, that is, time-intensive interactions between the doctor and the patient: careful history taking, care coordination, and preventive care. It would be better for the patients if insurance paid in a bundled fashion so that the incentive is to give good quality care along with good preventive care, as I discussed in chapter 8 regarding capitation and the large multi-specialty clinics.

A return to large risk pools is key. When you buy fire insurance for your home, you are part of a large risk pool, which helps keep down the cost for you. Our health-care risk pools are often too small. Most risk pools are based on your company. A company with relatively few employees has a small pool. If one person in that company has a truly catastrophic illness, such as the need for a bone marrow transplant or a kidney transplant, then that cost gets spread among those few employees in the next year's premiums. It is not a problem in a huge corporation where the risk is spread widely, but it becomes a real problem for a relatively small business. So the concept of an individual company being self-insured needs to disappear, and every company with an individual insurer should be part of a larger risk pool that will keep down the price. The argument against this approach would come from the company that institutes an effective wellness program, because if it is self-insured, the company's premiums will rise much more slowly as a result. That company wants to benefit financially from its efforts and not have it spread out over other companies that might not be as progressive and as effective.

Insurance should focus on catastrophic care. It is what insurance of all types traditionally covers. You pay a relatively small amount now so that in the unlikely event that you have a catastrophic fire in your house or you total your car, you will be reimbursed. Health-care insurance should also be for catastrophic care and not routine care. Then, as you do with auto collision insurance, you should be able to choose the level of deductible that you like. If you want a low deductible, you will pay a higher premium, and a higher deductible will make your premium correspondingly decline.

To be clear, medical insurance is still expensive, even when there is a high deductible so that it only pays for catastrophic needs. Chronic illnesses require more than a single hospitalization or surgical procedure; indeed, they are lifelong illnesses with recurring expenses that can and do add up. (By the way, that is why the Affordable Health Care Act included a provision to end "lifetime" caps on insurance coverage; you really need the coverage when a very catastrophic illness comes along.)

As has been previously discussed, the system has all sorts of other problems that keep high costs yet offer less-than-acceptable quality. We need to correct the system of care so that the cost of basic insurance plans can decline to more reasonable levels.

MEDICARE AND MEDICAID

Two other elements in our broken insurance system are Medicare and Medicaid. Medicare is an excellent program and, in fact, serves all of us who are older than sixty-five well. But the federal government consistently pays somewhat less than its full share of costs. The Medicare officials would say that limiting their reimbursement in effect forces hospitals to work hard to reduce the costs of medical care. This assertion is true to a degree, but the payment always seems to be less than what the hospitals bear as a cost. What happens with the balance? Other payers cross-subsidize the services. A large insurance company, such as Blue Cross/Blue Shield, usually is able to negotiate a rate with the hospital that is fairly close to the Medicare rate. But the smaller insurance company pays a somewhat higher rate, and that difference helps to make up for the losses with Medicare. The people who are uninsured and pay out of their own pocket pay the most. Indeed, self-paying patients, if they actually pay their full bill, end up paying upward of 300 percent of what Medicare pays for exactly the same service. This cross subsidization is a major issue. It results in increased costs to commercial insurers, and they pass those costs on to businesses such as your employer or to individuals like you. Basically this system is unfair, and it is a nationwide disaster. (Worth noting: If we had a single-payer plan such as Medicare for all, would no hospital or physician be paid in full for any patient?)

Medicaid is traditionally even worse as a payer than Medicare is. Medicaid usually pays well below what other insurers do. Hospitals might not like it, but they are generally expected to accept all patients and charge off the losses to charity care. It is illegal not to accept patients because they cannot pay or because they are on Medicaid. In fact, what really happens is that a hospital may try to find ways legally to discourage Medicaid patients from being admitted or from using its outpatient facilities. Doctors often refuse to take Medicaid patients because the rates are so low. Physicians have traditionally accepted everyone who comes to their door, recognizing that some could not pay or could not pay the full amount, but when the numbers of such patients become too great, the physicians tend to stop accepting Medicaid patients.

It is another reason why many specialists no longer will take emergency room duty. It was OK if the occasional patient was uninsured or on Medicaid, but with so many people now using the ER as their physician, the specialist feels he or she is unfairly burdened. Health-care reform places many more people on the Medicaid rolls, a laudable social good, but I doubt it will solve the ER problem. These people will have difficulty finding a PCP, so they will still go to the ER and the specialist will still be frustrated at the low reimbursement.

Medicare is generally good as an insurance system, but it does not cover the full costs of most services. It is worth pointing out that Medicare is neither cheap nor simple. As discussed in chapter 7, Medicare Part A, which is basically a hospital insurance policy, is free to everyone beginning at age sixty-five. ("Free" is a misnomer. In actuality you and your employer combined paid 2.9 percent [this amount has varied over time] of your earned income into the Medicare Trust Fund each year during your working lifetime. Add it up, include a reasonable factor for investment growth, and you may find that it is a fair sum of money. You paid for the coverage, but the system works differently. Your prior investment mostly covered the care of your parents. Once you start drawing on Medicare, it is being funded by your children's continuing Medicare tax payments.)

The government pays for half of Part B, or physician coverage, out of general tax revenues, and the policyholder pays the other half out of his or her Social Security check each month. Currently, this amount is $1,200 per year for most people. (The cost is more if your income is more than $85,000 if single and more than $170,000 if married.) But Part A and B do not cover everything, so most people buy what is known as a wraparound, or Medigap, policy from a private insurer. The federal government sets certain standards for these supplemental policies and what they must cover, ranging from the most basic (Plan A) to the broadest coverage (Plan L). Each insurer sets its own rates, but Plan A today might cost about $1,200 and Plan F, which can come with or without a high deductible, costs about $1,800 per year for someone who is between sixty-five and seventy years old. Finally, the newest addition is Part D, or drug coverage. It is provided through private insurers, with the individual paying a portion (about $360–625 per year) and the government paying a portion. When all the associated costs are added together for each person—$1,200 for Medicare Part B, $1,200 for the Medigap Plan A (or more if a more expensive Medigap policy is chosen), and $625 for Part D—a couple can easily be paying about $6,000 a year or more for coverage. That sum is a great deal of money considering that most people paid into Medicare all the years they were working. Calculate it out, and you will realize that you paid in a lot of money over your working career. It is still a good value; my point is only that Medicare is not "free."

Medicare, as with all health insurance policies, requires much paperwork. On the surface, it sounds smooth and simple, but for the physician and the hospital, an enormous amount of documentation must be submitted in order to get paid. Physicians are always anxious that their medical records will be audited to see if they can document that the level of care they claimed was actually provided. And the system is slow. It becomes really difficult if the patient is the one who sends in the forms to Medicare.

For example, my wife went to her physician to get the new herpes zoster, or shingles, vaccine. She had recently turned sixty-five and was on Medicare. The receptionist indicated that since Medicare almost certainly would not pay for it, the physician's office expected patients to pay for the shot up front (about $220, or $200 for the vaccine and $20 for getting the shot from the doctor) and then bill Medicare directly. The physician's office did not want to be saddled with the hassle of sending in the bill, having it rejected, trying another time, having it rejected again, and then finally having to bill the patient.

So my wife got the shot, paid for it, and then asked for a form to send into Medicare. The physician's office said it did not have that kind of form, but my wife could go to the Medicare website and download one. No such form was available online, so she called Medicare. After calling twice and being put on hold for a total of sixty-one minutes, someone answered and said, "Well, your physician should have billed for you, and if not they certainly should have given you the form!" My wife asked the person to send the form to her anyway. She finally received and sent in the form. Both Medicare and her Medigap wraparound policy rejected the claim for the vaccine, but she was reimbursed $20 toward the cost of its administration by the physician.

I am not suggesting that Medicare should or should not cover the zoster vaccine, (although I think it is a very valuable vaccine for an older person to get, as I wrote in *The Future of Medicine*), but I am arguing that the system does not work well. It should neither be that complex for the patient to figure out nor be so burdensome for the physician or the physician's office that physicians and their staffs do not want to be involved.

It turns out that there is more to my wife's story. Some months later we received in the mail new booklets about our benefits under the drug plan, or Part D. I usually file this material away, but I read it and found that the zoster vaccine was covered. I called the toll-free number, and although initially I was told that the zoster vaccine was not covered, I persisted. I gave the pharmacist on the phone the page number of the booklet that specified that it was covered. After some time, she came back on the line, stating that I was correct and that the company would pay, minus the co-pay. She sent a form by e-mail; we printed it and sent it in with the required proof of purchase and price. Soon a letter arrived that the bill was denied owing to "duplicate coverage," apparently meaning that we had been covered under Medicare and Medigap. But we had the denials from Medicare and from Medigap. We resent them, a few weeks later someone called to tell us that the claim had been approved and a check was forthcoming. Great! But when it came, it was for $142.18. It had been discounted by more than the co-pay, although the actual cost for the physician to buy the vaccine was $190. Some payment was better than nothing, but consider all the time, frustration, and bother we encountered.

Here is another example of the inefficiencies in Medicare and Medigap. My wife and I made the decision when we reached age sixty-five to purchase Plan F for our Medigap policy. It is the most expensive policy available through Blue Cross/ Blue Shield in Maryland, but we decided it was worth it for us. Given that my physician decided to begin retainer-based medicine a few years ago (see chapter 1), we also decided to change our Medigap policy to a high deductible. Our agent e-mailed us the forms, which we filled out and mailed to CareFirst Blue Cross/Blue Shield (CF). After a few weeks CareFirst sent us a letter saying that we had used the wrong form and asked if we would please fill out the new form that was enclosed. We did and mailed it back on December 2, 2008, but on December 24 we received new letters asking that we fill out a new set of forms as soon as possible. So we filled out the new ones and mailed them back. We looked at the forms closely and found that the only difference was the location on the form where we had to write in our names and addresses. The information was exactly the same, of course, but the box was slightly different. For this minor change, they wasted money and time in mailing us the forms. Multiply that process by a few or many thousand policyholders, and real money is wasted.

Medicare and commercial insurers should begin with the approach that both doctors and hospitals are inherently honest in their submissions. Certainly fraud and abuse occur and some bad apples try to bilk the system, so insurers need to have systems in place to uncover and stop them. But there is no reason that the systems need to be so complex, so difficult, so challenging, and, frankly, so frustrating for all concerned. Having a universal billing form would be a good start. Today every insurer requires a different form. Second, if all of us have a basic level of insurance with a high deductible (and were cared for in a true system of care), it should be possible to eliminate all denials, all resubmissions, and all the other techniques that insurers use either to slow the payment process or to deny payment for a service. Third, physicians and hospitals should be paid promptly, which would free up a good deal of working capital. Doctors and hospitals then could eliminate huge numbers of people who are currently employed simply to bill and verify claims. It would be much better if the system's dollars were used for patient care and not for administrative frustrations.

Here is an example of a physician carrying working capital to account for slow payments by insurers. My wife saw a physician in the fall of 2007. His office promptly sent in the Medicare forms for payment. In January 2009 she received a statement from Medigap that neither Medicare nor Medigap covered the visit, and she was responsible for the payment. But in the same mail came a separate letter from Medigap saying that the payment was approved. So which letter counts? When we looked at the forms carefully, the doctor's bill of $86 was reduced to $51 and then discounted further to $28. I can safely surmise that his overhead was more than the payment amount; he lost money seeing my wife. Of course, at the time we did not know if the letter that approved the bill or the one that rejected the bill would be the eventual final result. And if Medigap does pay the paltry amount approved, by law, the doctor cannot ask my wife to pay the balance. No wonder so many physicians would prefer not to participate in Medicare.

And indeed, they are choosing not to do so. My wife's PCP sent out a letter in 2010 stating, among other changes, that she would no longer be accepting Medicare. It is another of those disruptive changes spreading across the country. In my mind, it might be OK because my wife will pay directly for basic care. In return, she will expect prompt appointments, whatever time she needs per visit, and the ability to discuss carefully any recommendations for tests and procedures. And that was her experience in the first year of the new arrangement. But, on the negative side, it is a new expense because she still has (and needs) Medicare Part B and Medigap for all other physicians' visits, hospitalizations, or laboratory tests.

I happened to talk to the doctor after she had been using the new system of directly billing her patients for about six months. She told me that she now could give what she felt was really good care to lesser number of patients and that she felt much less hassled. She decided to go the next step and switched to the retainer-based model in July of 2011. She no longer needs a billing clerk to interact with the insurers.

Some real efforts to improve the system of insurance and especially its claims aspect could substantially affect health-care costs. Given all these frustrations, however, it follows that no single government payer should be created to take care of all Americans as the system has trouble handling Medicare claims now. Medicare does not pay full costs, which drives providers away, and this system actually amplifies the two classes of care that exist today.

As to commercial insurance, individuals should own their own health-care policy, not the employer. In this system, individuals would carry their policies with them from job to job or even when they didn't have a job. Losing coverage would no longer be an issue if they changed or lost their jobs. (The health-care reform bill prevents an insurer from refusing to cover someone with a preexisting condition.)

direct supplier ~ customer relationship ~ no distortion

This proposal does not mean that employers should no longer offer to pay for health insurance; rather, it means that individuals cannot be denied coverage because they leave one job and have a preexisting condition.

I mentioned the cross subsidization that occurs and how it drives up the costs for everybody else. The state of Maryland has a system that avoids this type of cross subsidy. It is called an all-payer system because by law each insurer must pay the same rate for the same hospital service. The state has created a commission called the Health Services Cost Review Commission that sets rates for each of the hospitals in the state. Once those rates are set, they are what everyone—including Medicare, Medicaid, CareFirst Blue Cross/Blue Shield, commercial insurers, and individuals—pays. In setting the rate, the commission includes a reasonable but not excessive markup over costs. This markup allows for the capital reinvestment in plant and technology that is critical to every hospital. The commission also includes an amount for uncompensated care in the rate for each hospital. Since different hospitals serve different populations, some hospitals have more uncompensated care than others do, and their rates will vary accordingly. As a result, those patients without insurance can access any hospital in the state and be assured of getting the same care as anyone else. (However, because the commission does not cover doctors' charges, physicians may or may not choose to accept patients who cannot pay.) Also, the commission-set rates include a medical education allowance, meaning that the expenses related to training residents, or the next generation of physicians, are included in the rates. So the basic result is that resources are equitably distributed across the hospitals in the state of Maryland.

Meanwhile, providers across the country have no incentive to be more effective or efficient, except where insurance does not reimburse for care, such as cosmetic surgery or Lasik eye surgery. The providers of these services compete on the basis of price and satisfaction, with prices coming down and satisfaction going up. Lasik surgery is a good example of the benefit of competition. As more ophthalmologists obtained the equipment and the training and offered the service, the prices declined rather dramatically over about five years. To get patient referrals for their service, the providers needed to offer the proper care and in a manner that satisfied customers. This example demonstrates the value of a direct financial relationship between the provider and the patient. In another, Wal-Mart sells inexpensive generic drugs for its customers. Basically, Wal-Mart is competing not only with the other pharmacies but also with the insurer by offering the drug for a price below the insurer's required co-pay.

Today's insurance, whether government or commercial, basically dampens entrepreneurship and competition in medical delivery. The care providers don't reap any benefit from doing the work for less; indeed, they are simply paid less. Instead, we need a system where providers could reap a greater profit in return for lowering the cost of care while maintaining quality. Everyone—the insurer (and its payer, which might be the individual, the employer, or the taxpayer), the providers, and the patients—would benefit in this new system.

Good care coordination will improve the quality of care for the individual patient yet will reduce costs by eliminating excess visits, tests, and procedures and by reducing the need for hospitalizations. Likewise, good preventive care will lower the total costs of care over an extended time. With primary care physicians not able or willing to take the necessary time with their patients today, clearly the system needs to find a way to coordinate care for those with complex, chronic illness and to offer preventive care to everyone. Insurers need to try various models or experiment to find systems that will improve the quality of care by ensuring both preventive care and care coordination while reducing the costs of care overall. Here is what one insurer, CareFirst Blue Cross/Blue Shield of Maryland; Washington, D.C.; and portions of Virginia, is considering.

CareFirst knows that about 80 percent of its medical expenditures go toward the care of 15–20 percent of its enrollees, or those patients who have catastrophic and complex, chronic illnesses. CareFirst also knows that primary care physicians receive about 5 percent of the total health-care expenditures yet PCPs are in a position to impact the other 95 percent of expenditures (i.e., for specialists, tests, procedures, and hospitalizations). So the CareFirst agenda is to create incentives for the PCPs to do so in a way that reduces that total while improving the care of the patient. The plan would work in the following (somewhat oversimplified) manner.

PCPs would form into virtual groups of five to ten people and enter into an agreement with CareFirst. In return CareFirst would increase their reimbursement by 15 percent for every visit and another 5 percent increment for using an electronic system provided by CareFirst that will assist with billing. This system will check their submissions, make edits and corrections, and then submit the claim to CareFirst (or any insurer), all automatically and electronically. I am told it is easy to use and will greatly improve the doctor's office productivity, thus creating savings. No longer will claims be denied over billing errors or the need to repeatedly resubmit until the claim is remediated, because it will be correct the first time. In addition, CareFirst will agree to pay the physician within one business day, dramatically reducing the need for working capital.

CareFirst will conduct an analysis of the PCP group's patients using claims data from the prior year. CareFirst will be able to flag the 15–20 percent or so of those patients who need care coordination. The PCP's obligation in this new system is to give the patient whatever added time is needed per visit, create a good care plan, and post it in an electronic medical record. This care plan will serve as automatic pre-authorization; therefore, the PCP will not need to make any further calls to CF for tests, procedures, and so on, resulting in another major timesaver for the PCP and his or her office staff. When the patient needs to see a specialist, the PCP will refer the patient, will call the specialist to clarify expectations, and will review the results of the referral. Finally, CareFirst will make available a care coordinator (a nurse) to call the patient as often as necessary to check on medication use, medication side effects, weight gain, or other factors that the PCP has built into the care plan. If the care coordinator cannot resolve an issue or sees a problem developing, she or he will report it to the PCP. The expectation is that this approach of incentives for the PCP's giving the patient the required care coordination will enhance the quality while reducing the overall expenditures for that patient's care.

Adding to the incentives, CareFirst will do an actuarial analysis of the expected claims for the coming year for the PCP group's patients. If, at the end of the year, the patients have had fewer claims, CF will give back a portion of its savings through higher reimbursements to the PCPs. With this additional incentive, it is anticipated that the PCPs will be sure to coordinate care scrupulously so that there are no excess specialist visits, no unneeded tests or procedures, and, with better care overall, fewer hospitalizations. The end results, hopefully, will be higher quality care, lower total expenditures for that care, enhanced income for the PCPs, and a more satisfying practice. It could be a win for everyone. Of course, the devil is in the details of how it is actually implemented, but it seems to be a worthy plan, one that might have a real impact. This approach appeals to me because it begins with an attempt to improve quality as a means of reducing costs rather than starting with arbitrary cost reductions.

The care coordination described here is a major part of the contemplated CareFirst Blue Cross/Blue Shield plan. But three other components are key. First, the plan will provide better care at a lower cost. The PCP will receive increased compensation for seeing all patients, not only for those with complex, chronic illnesses.

Hopefully, this greater payment will be enough to ensure that every patient gets the time and attention needed for the best possible care from the physician. It also should mean that the PCP will be less inclined to refer a patient to a specialist quickly rather than taking the time needed to sort out the patient's problem first. By the same logic, it is anticipated that if the physician takes a more complete history and performs a more thorough physical exam, it will negate the need for more tests and procedures. It will result in better care for the patient, who will be more satisfied because the doctor will not be in a rush, and in a more satisfied physician because he or she is being compensated for the extra time to give better care.

Next, CareFirst recognizes that more than 90 percent of its clients remain with CF year after year, so financially it is logical to try to ensure good preventive care. This effort will cost more today, but the investment should pay off in the years to come with lower costs because the client will remain healthy. So in this new practice arrangement, CareFirst will pay for any preventive measure, screening program, and test that is well defined by evidence. This service might include cholesterol measurements, mammography and colonoscopy, and dietary consultation or a smoking cessation program. As an added incentive to get this type of preventive care done, CF will waive any co-pays or deductibles that the patient might have to otherwise pay.

Finally, it is recognized that some small percentage of patients will develop a truly catastrophic condition for which the PCPs will no longer be able to coordinate the care easily. These patients, who might need major surgery or perhaps an organ transplant, will have to be referred to a specialty center or an academic medical center. My own observations over the years demonstrate that these types of patients receive less than the best possible care because the handoffs and referrals among providers are less than satisfactory. These transitions are when quality breaks down, safety issues arise, and all too often excessive tests and procedures are done. Since no one is orchestrating the entire care program, the patient is left with well-intentioned caregivers but less than the best care.

In this situation, CareFirst will develop an incentive-based relationship with the specialty provider—probably a hospital system—to ensure continuing care coordination. To each patient the hospital system will assign a navigator who will have the responsibility of ensuring that the patient's care within the system is well coordinated, just as the PCP does in the community setting. This navigator will work the interface among the myriad specialists, departments, and even hospitals and centers that the patient must use for his or her care. CareFirst hopes that the result should be much better care quality yet at a substantially reduced total cost.

The whole CareFirst contemplated concept is to coordinate the care that the patient receives with the expectation that the patient will be better served, the providers will be more satisfied, and the total costs will be reduced. It will mean a real change in how the system works. The primary care physician will evolve from being an intervener to being an orchestrator who offers effective preventive care. The hospital system will become an orchestrator as well and not simply be a place for specialty care. And this model represents a change for the insurer, too. It accepts that care coordination and preventive care cost money now, that streamlining the claims submission process will result in reduced costs for the physician, and that the end result is better care at a lower total cost.

REHABILITATION, SUB-ACUTE CARE, HOME CARE, AND HOSPICE CARE

Other factors need to be adjusted as a result of this shift from handling acute problems to those of long-term and chronic illnesses. For one, our current reimbursement systems are fundamentally based on acute care because most of the insurance systems were created when acute care was the predominant situation. But our reimbursement system and care needs have changed with the rise of complex, chronic conditions.

Frequently, a patient must leave the general hospital and go to a rehabilitation center after suffering a trauma or a stroke, for example. Rehabilitation care is much less expensive than general hospital care is, and fortunately most insurance policies will pay for a reasonable stay in the rehabilitation hospital if it is appropriate. Also, the patient with a long-term, complex illness needs coverage for outpatient physical therapy as a follow-up to that stay at the rehabilitation hospital; for sub-acute care in a less intensive area of the hospital with a lower staffing ratio to prepare the patient's transition to functioning at home; for home care, which essentially means that a nurse stops by the home on a regular basis to assist the patient; and for hospice care.

We need a system of care and a reimbursement system that accepts and encourages good rehabilitation care, sub-acute care, home care, and hospice care. It will reduce the total expenditures while much improving the quality of care and quality of life for the individual and his or her family. A step in the right direction may be in the reform legislation (Affordable Health Care Act), which specifically will establish a national, voluntary, bundled payment pilot program for acute care hospitals and post-acute care providers. Bundled payments could encourage acute and post-acute care providers to work together by aligning incentives.

Finally, although we should not consider the insurers blameless, it is not appropriate to blame solely them for the high costs of medical care today. The insurers, as we have seen, are largely third-party payers who collect from the employer (or individual) and use the funds to pay the providers. If the providers use large amounts of visits, procedures, tests, drugs, and hospitalizations to treat their patients, then the costs of care will be high and the resulting costs of insurance will rise. Basically, the insurers pass on the costs they are confronting. The real need is to find ways to bring down the actual costs by improving care coordination, augmenting preventive care, and incentivizing the patients with high-deductible policies to become actively involved in their care decisions.

13

The Looming Crisis in Primary Care

Misconception: *Primary care physicians do not deal with the expensive aspects of medical care so they can have little impact on reducing medical expenditures.*

An elderly immigrant, Sophia, and her daughter had been seeing the same primary care physician for more than twenty years. She lived in another city about thirty miles distant, but she preferred to visit the doctor with her daughter because of her language concerns. She also occasionally saw a doctor near her home if she had an immediate problem. During nearly every visit Sophia said that she felt "tired." Repeated histories, exams, and logical tests such as those for anemia and hypothyroidism revealed no cause. She then developed syncopal episodes, times when she would black out, fall to the floor (once bruising her head when she fell against the stove), and then wake up in a few minutes. The PCP's evaluation showed that she had intermittent episodes of bradycardia, or very slow heart rate, resulting in the drop attacks. In consultation with a cardiologist, it was decided to insert a single-lead, "demand" pacemaker. The pacemaker is implanted under the skin on the upper chest and a wire, or lead, is tunneled under the skin to a vein in the neck and from there into the heart, where it is positioned against the wall of the ventricle. The pacemaker senses the electrical action in the heart, and when the rate drops below a set level, it sends an electrical stimulus, on demand, to the heart muscle so that it will contract at a normal speed or rate. The pacemaker and the procedure to place it are expensive, but it worked perfectly. Sophia no longer had the attacks that were not only scary but seriously impacting her quality of life. She had a good return on her investment.

A few months later, when Sophia went to the internist in her hometown for an unrelated reason, he urged her to see a cardiologist colleague of his near her home.

The cardiologist, in turn, recommended that she needed a dual-lead pacemaker instead of the single-lead one she had. (It has been found that having more than one lead can sometimes improve the heart's output for carefully selected patients with heart failure.) Sophia's daughter reported this recommendation to the longtime PCP who noted that her mother did not have heart failure, but syncopal attacks. Further, the current pacemaker was only needed about 10 percent of the time, meaning that her heart beat at a normal rate at least 90 percent of the time, so the pacemaker was not even active most of the day. They quickly agreed that Sophia did not need the proposed new, highly expensive pacemaker. A great deal of money was saved and the patient was spared a straightforward yet somewhat risky procedure and the risks involved with insertion or postoperative infection or bleeding.

Why did the cardiologist suggest the dual-lead pacemaker? Because, as always, the patient had reported that she was tired. He had interpreted this complaint as possibly meaning heart failure and thought that the extra oomph of the dual-lead pacemaker would give her more energy. While it is an interesting theory, if he had been more thorough in his history taking or had called the PCP, the cardiologist would have realized that Sophia's problem was not new and didn't need to be resolved technologically. Once the PCP became aware of the issue and intervened, an unnecessary procedure and device were avoided. (A less charitable theory is that the cardiologist stood to benefit substantially from doing a procedure but not from a simple consult visit.)

The lesson here is one doctor needs to be the orchestrator of all of the patient's care. A good PCP, like this one, coordinates the care of his or her patients with chronic illnesses and in so doing avoids excess referrals, tests, procedures, and hospitalizations along with unneeded drugs or devices—all elements that drive up the total cost of care. In the process, care coordination ensures quality care, safer care, and a close doctor-patient relationship.

One of the most effective ways to reduce medical care costs is with good coordination of the care of individuals with chronic illnesses. As Sophia's story and as Henry's story from chapter 8 exemplify, there is a strong tendency for patients to be referred to various specialists or else they go on their own. When these visits occur without coordination, the visits add up, the number of tests and images ordered increase, the number of drugs prescribed rises rapidly, and the number of procedures and even hospitalizations climb. Unfortunately, many are simply not needed; indeed, they are excessive and wasteful, not the best quality, and obviously very costly.

The primary care physician is in the best position to coordinate care. He or she knows the patient, the patient's family and socio-economic situation, and, of course, the patient's medical history. Sophia did not need to see a second cardiologist and did not need the dual-lead pacemaker. The PCP knew that "tired" was her normal report at every visit; it was not a reason to do more tests, add a drug, or perform a new procedure. It was unfortunate, indefensible, but not at all uncommon that the new cardiologist did not make the effort to call Sophia's longtime PCP. Even though they practiced thirty miles apart, the cardiologist knew the PCP, and they actually shared a few patients. Indeed, the cardiologist had the PCP's personal cell phone number. One call would have quickly determined that she did not need an expensive new pacemaker. Fortunately, the PCP became aware of the recommendation and intervened.

Henry suffered because he did not have a primary care physician. Instead he saw four doctors, each one dealing with all of his problems but not communicating with the other providers. When he began seeing a single PCP, his prescriptions plummeted from twenty-three to seven, he felt better, and he had fewer drug-induced side effects. Moreover, both he and his insurer (a private insurer through Medicare Part D) were saving a great deal of money.

Today, many if not most PCPs do not take much time to coordinate care of chronic illnesses or deal with prevention. They administer a few shots and write a prescription here and there, but they do not spend any real time in counseling and carefully assessing the patient's preventive health needs. Why? The reasons are many, but in the end it comes down to dollars and cents. Briefly stated, PCPs feel overwhelmed with paperwork, find they must see ever more patients to maintain a level income, and are gradually losing more of their family time. The result is fewer individuals are entering primary care, fewer still work in underserved areas, more PCPs are retiring early, and more and more they are looking for ways either to exit entirely or to find a more rational approach to practice. They want a practice that they can be proud of and an income commensurate with their expertise and competence, yet still have time for family and friends. The following story may help explain the situation better.

I have known Dr. Robert Miller for more than thirty years. He went to one of the best medical schools, did an excellent internal medicine program for three years, and spent an additional two years in subspecialty training, including another two years at the National Institutes of Health. In his early thirties, he started his primary care internal medicine practice in a growing suburban community and quickly became well recognized for his careful, attentive, and collaborative manner. His practice grew. He enjoyed caring for patients and soon partnered with two other physicians who were recently out of their training programs. In general, a claim submitted to an insurance company was paid in full and promptly. Office staff was minimal. Over time and as his practice developed, his income, adjusted for today's dollars, grew to about $150,000 annually. He and his partners shared night and weekend calls and eventually added a few additional physicians, making being on call even less burdensome. They always met their patients at the emergency room and cared for them in the local hospital. They spent the time necessary to ensure that each patient received appropriate attention, and they tried to address all the preventive and screening issues. Each of them also gave free medical time to the community. They each recognized that not everyone was financially fortunate and accepted patients who could not pay or could not pay fully.

As time went on, practice became increasingly difficult. The insurers' requirements became burdensome at best, and the doctors needed more staff to process claims and to seek preapprovals for computed tomography scans, for referrals to specialists, and for elective hospitalizations. The insurers negotiated rates that at best were flat from year to year, always saying that the doctors were receiving competitive payments. The low government payment rates (primarily Medicare for Dr. Miller) then became the benchmark for the commercial insurers as well. The group's office expenses were rising, the workload was increasing, and in order to maintain their own income at a flat level, the doctors had to see more patients per day. Robert could not bear to tell his patients that their "time was up," so he would have his nurse knock on the examining room door and say it was time to move on. He felt he was no longer able to have quality interaction with his patients, for he did not have the time to learn about his patients' personal and family situation. He had particularly enjoyed that part of the dialogue and felt that it made him a better doctor. As a way to create more office time, they stopped attending to their hospitalized patients; instead, they turned them over to the hospital-employed hospitalists. Often they did not go to the ER but simply called in and waited to hear the emergency medicine physician's assessment by phone. They also found there was too little time to coordinate care for those with chronic illnesses, or calling each specialist and explaining the patient's situation and the reason for the referral. And they had all too little time actually to sit with a patient and explain basic preventives measures. Most importantly, there was little time to just "think."

Eventually, the group became so frustrated that it decided to make a major change. The doctors knew that some of their local colleagues in primary care had contracted with various vendors and allowed them to do tests and procedures in their office space. (For example, some let vendors perform heart stress tests in their offices and collected a fee even though the results were still reviewed by an outside cardiologist later.) They were not comfortable with this concept. They had explored an annual "administrative" charge but had been told it was not acceptable with their various insurance carrier contracts, including Medicare. Some other local primary care physicians had signed up with MDVIP, a network of physicians that use the retainer-based arrangement. Eventually they decided to make the leap and go with retainer-based care. It meant that they would reduce the number of patients that they cared for from about fifteen hundred patients each to about five hundred. Each of the remaining patients would pay an annual fee and receive unlimited visits, each for as much time as the doctor and patient felt was necessary. The doctors promised to be available by cell phone 24/7, to meet a patient at the ER, to care for the patient in the hospital, to make home or nursing home visits as needed, to respond to e-mails, and to do whatever else seemed necessary for their patients. In short, they were going back to the practice they had had many years before. But everything has its trade-offs, and one was the anger and frustration of those who chose not to participate and pay the annual retainer. Some felt it represented greed, and a few wrote letters to the local paper. Even those who did buy in were upset that on top of their insurance premiums they now had an additional monetary burden.

We are appropriately fascinated with the medical miracles brought to us largely through specialists. But the backbone of the medical care system (and the hoped for, true health-care system) is the primary care physician. To correct our system and have it work properly for all, we need PCPs in adequate numbers providing good preventive care and good care coordination. Absent PCPs performing these functions, medical costs will continue to rise, and rise fast. In addressing these escalating costs, we should focus on the PCPs and their role in health care. This is the place to put the emphasis on action. In my opinion, it is fortunate that we still have at least some practicing PCPs, and that many of them have decided to reassert their right to provide appropriate care and to be appropriately compensated in return. Let's look at this in some detail.

BACKGROUND TO THE PRESENT PROBLEM

Medicare began in the mid-1960s and introduced a different dynamic for paying physicians. First, and very important, the patient no longer paid the physician directly; instead, payment came from the government. Patients, as a result, no longer cared what the services cost. As costs rose, and they rose much faster than anyone in government had anticipated, Medicare looked for ways to get control. In 1992, Medicare introduced the Resource-Based Relative Value Scale (RBRVS) to determine the payments for various services. Although an objective system, it is inherently tilted in favor of specialists, especially those who do procedures or do surgery. Further, there are no payment codes for services such as reviewing an e-mail, spending time on prevention counseling, or taking time to coordinate the care of a patient with a chronic illness such as heart failure. The result over time, as commercial insurers followed Medicare's lead, is a system in which PCPs receive proportionately less and less compensation for their services.

An important element came later with the congressionally mandated sustainable growth rate calculation. Basically payments for all physician services are a zero-sum game. If expenditures are up for all physicians' services, then Medicare fees are to be reduced across the board for all providers. But since the reasons for the increased expenditures are more visits to specialists and uses of tests and imaging, the PCP ends up with a relatively greater reduction in Medicare payments. Commercial insurers tend to rapidly follow Medicare's lead and even exacerbate this differential.

The result over time has been a huge widening of the income gap between generalists and specialists. Medical students, like everyone else, look around and make economic decisions in choosing their career directions, and fewer and fewer graduates enter primary care. Meanwhile, generalists in current practice at least want to maintain their current income and preferably would like to see it keep pace with inflation. Receiving less income per patient encounter, their response has been to increase the number of patients they see. It is the old economic response to reduced price: try to make it up with volume. To accomplish this aim, they must extend their office hours or shorten visit times or both. Most PCPs also stop attending their patients in the hospital or in the ER, thereby creating time for more office visits. And shorter visits have become the unfortunate norm.

But PCPs (and all physicians) are also frustrated by other elements of the current insurance system. They are beset with increased regulations and workload to get preauthorization, to collect co-pays and deductibles, to bill and to rebill and to rebill the insurer. At some point the combination of lower payments, increased frustration, and excessive workload—a workload that the physician knows is not ideal for his or her patients or for himself or herself—leads to a decision to change the approach to reimbursement or to close the practice and seek employment with a hospital or other provider organization. So we have a decreasing number of graduates choose to become generalists, fewer physicians remain in classical private practice, and more and more physicians are either refusing to accept insurance or switching to retainer-based practices models.

SHORTAGE OF PRIMARY CARE PHYSICIANS

We have an inadequate number of primary care physicians or their equivalents. Most countries have about 70 percent or more of their physicians in primary care settings whereas the United States has about 70 percent working as specialists. This gradual transition to specialization over the past fifty years is largely because of our insurance system, which basically pays for a visit or a procedure. It results in less reward for the primary care doctor, who does few if any procedures.

We need a system that compensates the generalist in an appropriate manner. Today, the average general internal medicine practitioner earns about $150,000. It's not a bad income until you consider that he or she only started working at about age thirty-two (after college, medical school, residency, and possibly extra training in a fellowship), carries usually at least $100,000 of debt, and has long hours and an enormous responsibility (for your health!). That doctor's salary has remained stagnant for the past few years, despite the need for raises for the office staff, the rent, and the utilities. A starting internist or pediatrician or family medicine doctor can expect to earn about $80,000. No wonder they prefer to consider a specialty practice, where the income is higher but hardly high by today's standards for many lawyers, accountants, and other professionals. With demoralized physicians toiling in a non-sustainable business model, it is no wonder that only about a thousand graduates enter primary care each year while about three thousand to four thousand leave.

More and more medical school graduates choose to be employed by hospitals now rather than be part of a physician-owned practice. Traditionally most physicians have been in private practice; as recently as 2002 it amounted to about 75 percent.

Today that number has dropped to about 35 percent. During the same time period, hospital-employed physicians have risen from about 25 percent to nearly 60 percent. The reasons are clear. Physicians are simply fed up with wrangling with insurers, and being expected to collect co-pays and deductibles from their patients, and other frustrations. It is simpler to let the hospital serve all of these functions. In the end, the traditional contractual relationship between doctor and patients has been broken by our perverse insurance system.

Why is the United States so different with only 30 percent of doctors serving as PCPs? As stated previously, reimbursement mechanisms developed during the past fifty years or so created this disparity. Generalists' pay is typically much lower than is pay for specialists, usually by 50 percent or more. Those who do procedures, such as cardiologists and gastroenterologists, and those who do surgery generally tend to earn more than does a generalist who focuses on listening, prevention activities, and cognitive activities.

Incentives are needed to encourage graduates of medical schools to enter primary care fields, such as internal medicine, pediatrics, and family medicine. Part of the incentive package must be for spending time on prevention, counseling, and taking patient histories. In short, it means markedly improving reimbursement both for cognitive activities and for prevention, wellness, and health promotion visits. Further, the physician can only do this work if he or she has no more than about five hundred patients to care for and not twelve hundred or more.

Recall that the primary care physician in aggregate receives about 5 percent of the dollars spent on medical care, but the PCP is in a pivotal position to affect the other 95 percent of the dollars consumed. We need to create incentives so the PCP will assume the task of actually coordinating the other aspects of care. It will mean paying the PCP more—maybe increasing his or her "share" to about 6–7 percent—but the potential impact could be a major reduction in the total dollars spent. We would see a high return on our investment provided the PCP is given more funding (rights) only in return for actually being an orchestrator who manages the full coordination of care (responsibilities.) This major change will have a substantial impact but will take time to implement because the PCP will need to reduce his or her practice size and markedly rework his or her practice. This approach is much more effective than simply cutting the reimbursement rates (price) for specialists, which will create extreme ill will. Instead, if the PCP coordinates care, the specialist will get fewer referrals, the labs will conduct fewer tests, the radiologists will have fewer images to interpret, the drug companies will see fewer prescriptions for their highest priced drugs, and the hospitals will have fewer admissions. But because the population is aging and more illnesses will occur in the coming years, the specialists, labs, radiologists, drug companies, and hospitals will do fine in the long run. And, if this development leads to having too many specialists and to increased incomes for generalists, then more and more graduates will choose to become PCPs.

With or without a complex, chronic disease (or more than one), everyone needs good care coordination. Think of the primary care provider as the patient's general contractor. Just as the contractor organizes and monitors the carpenter, mason, electrician, and others, the PCP should be encouraged to organize and supervise all of the elements of the patient's care and be held responsible for ensuring that everyone does their part at the right time and the right place.

The message here is that the linchpin of health care is the primary care provider; thus, incentivizing PCPs of all types ultimately will reduce the cost of care in a beneficial fashion. To accomplish this mission, the primary care physician must shift from today's interventionalist to tomorrow's orchestrator. Other providers must be encouraged and, indeed, allowed to serve as appropriate. These proposals are major paradigm changes, and disruptive of today's practice patterns, but they need to occur and will occur only if the physicians and insurers are willing to make major changes. Each group will have to accept new rights and responsibilities to make it work. The result can be a substantial decrease in the cost of health care with big improvements in care quality and patient satisfaction. And I venture to say that the PCP will be happier as a result.

ADJUNCT PROVIDERS AND PRIMARY CARE

Practitioners other than physicians, such as nurse practitioners or physician's assistants (PAs), can offer substantial primary care, but the medical establishment frequently has done its darnedest to limit these individuals' activities, usually on the basis that such a practitioner simply does not have the knowledge base, the experience, or the credentials to take adequate care of patients. Ophthalmologists often oppose letting optometrists put drops in patients' eyes, psychiatrists try to place barriers around what a psychologist or social worker can do in their practice, and so on. The reasons given are always that the highly educated and trained physician is in a better position to care for a patient, but the real issue, of course, is the professional not wanting others to tramp on his or her turf. No, other practitioners do not have the same education or training and cannot perform at the same level that physicians do, but they are competent. There is a role for all of these practitioners, preferably while working with a physician who, in turn, needs to serve as the orchestrator of a team-based approach to care. But the important issue is that, besides the inadequate numbers of PCPs, the absence of alternative practitioners also reduces care quality and drives up health-care costs.

Physicians need to embrace the work of adjunct providers. These practitioners, such as nurse practitioners, physician assistants, and others, need to be encouraged to offer primary care; optometrists coaxed to offer primary eye care; and psychologists and social workers enticed to offer primary mental health care. Likewise, there need to be incentives for pharmacists to use their clinical training to do patient education and counseling, which can go a long way toward improving the use of medications, decreasing side effects, and improving compliance.

Another consideration relates to paramedics. When not on ambulance runs, they could assist with care coordination by calling patients to check on care plans. And with the proper added certification, and perhaps in telemedicine consultation with a physician as needed, they could care for many problems in a patient's home rather than taking the patient to the hospital or ER for expensive treatment. For example, a common call is for a dehydrated older person. If the paramedic could begin intravenous fluid hydration at the home or nursing home, the person might not need to be moved to the ER. Changing the regulations to allow the paramedic to administer some treatments would lead to better quality care and a big savings.

In late 2010 the Institute of Medicine issued a report urging changes that would maximize the education and expertise of nurses, including nurse practitioners. Among the IOM's recommendations was lifting the current various barriers that limit the work of nurses and advanced practice nurses such as NPs.

Many of us, but unfortunately not all of us, have a dentist we see twice per year. Dental care is an essential element of primary care. Maintaining healthy teeth is important, not only to prevent cavities, but also because they are critical for our short- and long-term health. Because they see their patients regularly, dentists can be the first ones to detect oral disease and other problems that should prompt a visit to a primary care provider.

It is important that all providers work together as a team. When they do, the outcome for patients is enhanced dramatically.

THE MEDICAL HOME AND ACCOUNTABLE CARE ORGANIZATIONS

There needs to be a fundamental overhaul of how primary care is delivered. The first requirement should be for form to follow function, meaning we should decide what the intended health-care function is and then, and only then, should we design the delivery system to meet it. Unfortunately, medical care has tended to work the other way, with systems being established and then being jerry-rigged to get the job done. Instead, we need to begin with the concept that the patient is a consumer who needs convenient, timely, reliable access to his or her provider(s). Often this access will mean an office visit, but it could be satisfied with a phone call, an e-mail exchange, or a telemedicine encounter using Skype as well. Today the visit or encounter is with the physician, but often it could be as effective with a nurse practitioner or other adjunct provider. When the generalist feels he or she needs a consult, today the patient is sent to a specialist; however, the problem often could be resolved on the spot with a virtual consultation using Skype or a more sophisticated technology.

For all of these changes to work, reimbursement models also need to be altered so that, here again, form follows the function. If the function is correct, then the payment (form) should apply. Old systems of insurance will change but slowly and with much effort; however, the reimbursement systems must change with it.[1]

With an appreciation that form must follow function, it will be possible to develop new models of care that respond to the needs for better preventive care and for well-coordinated care of those with chronic illnesses. The "patient-centered medical home" (PCMH) begins with the premise that excellent primary care is the bedrock of a good care system. The idea is to align the incentives (rights) and the accountabilities (responsibilities) across the entire care continuum. The PCMH combines continuous, comprehensive coordinated care with a good electronic medical record, continuous quality improvement, management of chronic illness, the liberal use of nonphysician providers—all to meet the needs and preferences of the patient and the patient's family. The difficulty of getting this PCMH model up and running is the current reimbursement system. Unless it changes, this great idea will be rarely implemented.

The health-care reform legislation, Affordable Care Act, mandates the creation of accountable care organizations (ACOs). The concept is that the organization, presumably provider led, will manage the full spectrum of care for a defined population. It is an outgrowth of managed care concepts in that the organization receives a fixed sum of money for the year for a large group of patients and becomes accountable for

Quality

Fixed Budget

the patients' health.[2] Since good preventive care, primary care, and care coordination will improve quality and reduce expenses, the providers are incented to deliver these services effectively.

By its very nature, an ACO will require a very strong foundation of integrated primary care. As with the PCMH, ACOs will only be effective if the payment system properly aligns incentives to improve the quality and safety of care as the fundamental goal. Cost savings must be an outgrowth, not the driving purpose, of the model.

PRIMARY CARE AND PREVENTION: MANAGEMENT OF DISEASE

When we think of the new medical care delivery system that the United States needs, it is critical to understand what works and why. We need to encourage patients to maximize the benefits of good care and to incentivize physicians and other providers to make the new medical care available to everyone at the right time and place.

All children should have access to each of the recommended immunizations. Vaccinations are incredibly cost-effective medicine. Critical screenings, easily done and not expensive, for vision, hearing, cholesterol, body mass index (BMI), and pulmonary function tests for asthma detection can be accomplished at the children's schools. When these problems are caught at a young age, intervention can have a lifetime of value and reduce potential negative impacts on long-term health-care expenditures. And in conjunction with these measures, each child needs a primary care provider who can be the child's caregiver and advocate over a long period.

Elderly individuals are, like children, the greatest beneficiaries of preventive care. They need insurance, presumably Medicare or a supplemental policy, that covers those critical elements of care delivery that enhance their well-being and keep them out of a nursing home with all of its financial costs, quality of life issues, and so on. Vision and hearing screening and remediation are first on the list, followed by psychological assistance for depression and anxiety and physical therapy or personal trainers to help with mobility. The elderly also need screening for blood pressure, blood sugar, and cholesterol, for it is never too late to prevent chronic illness. Screening for vitamin D levels is important because vitamin D is increasingly recognized as being essential for many bodily functions—not simply bone health—and most older Americans are deficient. Tax credits to build ramps to the front door, place grab bars in the bathroom, and install elevated toilets all encourage living at home rather than moving to a nursing home. The elderly also need continuing dental care if only to ensure good nutrition.

Social workers can assist with mental health and general support of the elderly patient. Complementary medical approaches such as acupuncture and massage for chronic pain can have valuable results. When a patient needs intravenous antibiotics for some period of time, this treatment at home costs less than hospitalization does, but often it is not covered. An added value of home-based antibiotic therapy is that the patient usually does not become disoriented, fall, and break an osteoporotic bone, as might occur in the hospital, and the patient won't develop a hospital-acquired secondary infection. Insurers should consider these factors when running a cost-benefit analysis to determine coverage. Insurance needs to take all of these factors into consideration. It is all about preventive care, which is generally inexpensive yet can have a big return of investment.

PAYING FOR COORDINATION AND PREVENTION

If PCPs are to give their patients quality preventive care and carefully coordinate chronic illnesses, they will need to adjust their schedules markedly and receive major changes in payments in return. As part of the Affordable Care Act, Medicare will soon raise its fees by 5–10 percent for primary care, but this amount will not be enough either to allow PCPs to lighten their patient load, or to encourage graduates to enter primary care fields. What needs to be done?

PCPs need to have no more than about five hundred active patients, and those serving mostly a geriatric population should have no more than about four hundred patients. (These numbers could go higher in a clinical setting where a PCP works with NPs, PAs, and so on, but it is essential that the PCP have adequate time with each patient and additional time for coordination work.) As noted previously, however, most PCPs today have twelve hundred patients or more. Each patient gets a short visit, there is no time for extensive conversation, it is easier to refer the patient to a specialist than to figure out the problem, and prescriptions are used instead of counseling. No longer do PCPs attend their patients in the hospital or meet them at the ER. (In fairness, some PCPs actually do all of these functions. They are to be commended, but unfortunately they are increasingly the minority.) E-mail could save time and office visits, but without reimbursement, PCPs generally refuse to give out their e-mail address.

In an effort to establish a more workable situation, many physicians now refuse to accept Medicare or commercial insurance. They ask their patients instead to pay a reasonable fee out of pocket. They also might ask for an annual fee for e-mail communication. This arrangement returns the doctor-patient relationship to an economic contractual one. If the patient feels the price is too high or the service insufficient, he or she can negotiate for a lower fee or better service or go to another doctor.

Retainer-Based Practices

A second approach to improving PCPs' working conditions and providing better care options is the retainer-based practice. As discussed previously, the patient pays the physician an annual retainer of $1,500 to $2,000 and in return is guaranteed that the physician will keep his or her practice to about five hundred patients total, be available 24/7 by e-mail and cell phone and for an office visit within twenty-four hours, will meet the patient at the ER when necessary, will make house calls and nursing home visits, and will attend the patient if hospitalized. This system really harks back to what the doctor-patient relationship used to be. Unstated, but essential if this style of care is to be useful, is the physician's promise truly to coordinate the care of chronic illnesses and to pay attention to preventive care. In effect it is a direct contract between the doctor and the patient in which each has certain rights and responsibilities. Absent a change in the way insurance pays for primary care, this setup may prove to be the best approach.

Many primary care internists are making this conversion, with numbers rising from about five hundred in 2005 to five thousand in 2009 and an estimated twenty thousand in 2012. These estimates are substantially more that the Medicare Payment Advisory Commission found in its report in late 2010.[3] Whatever the exact numbers, they are rising quickly. I predict that more and more PCPs will opt for this approach. For them, it allows for the delivery of better care in a less hectic environment with far fewer hassles with insurers. But the real beneficiary is the patient, who now has both a direct contractual relationship and, most important, a doctor who has the time to provide much better care. Of course, it should not have transpired this way. Our insurance should have always paid the PCP an adequate amount for appropriate care so that the doctor would have the time needed to be effective and thorough.

Direct Payment for Primary Care

Perhaps the best alternative, since it is unlikely that insurance will ever pay appropriately, would be for all of us to accept the notion we have to pay our doctors directly. General and routine care such as annual exams, vaccinations, and preventive screening could be paid for out of pocket; more expensive yet unanticipated costs could be paid for with savings in a health savings account; and only very expensive or catastrophic care could be paid for with insurance. This plan also returns the doctor and the patient to a classic financial contractual relationship. It is clear who the client is, namely, the recipient of the service. Of course, not everyone can afford these basics, so the government would still need to assist them. This assistance could be in the form of vouchers or a tax credit, still allowing the patient to have a direct contractual relationship with the physician.

DISEASE MANAGEMENT AND PRIMARY CARE OVERSIGHT

I will be somewhat repetitive here but intentionally so to emphasize a point. Let's shift gears and look at the problem that has developed as medicine has converted from largely treating acute problems such as pneumonia and appendicitis to such chronic, complex problems as diabetes with complications, chronic kidney disease, or heart failure. Indeed, about 70–80 percent of medical costs are expended on the 10–15 percent of patients who have these types of chronic, complex illnesses. We desperately need a change in the way we reimburse caregivers so that we can have real care management programs, programs that are focused on treating disease rather than being built around a specialty, team-based care, and improved payments for the time generalists spend with patients in cognitive activities such as history taking and counseling. In chapter 6, for example, I introduced the Joslin Diabetes Center concept. The center is built on the concept that the patient with diabetes requires the expertise of many different individuals and that those individuals need to be readily available, all at the same location, and working together as a team. This center makes it easy for the patient to get from caregiver to caregiver, for the caregivers to communicate one with another, and, when a problem arises, for the patient to have it quickly addressed.

Consider team care or disease management for a patient with heart failure. Heart failure occurs often after one or more heart attacks have damaged the muscle of the heart so that it cannot pump as strongly as before. Most patients who have heart attacks today survive and do fine, but a certain proportion develop heart failure. Indeed, there is actually an "epidemic" of heart failure today in America. Heart failure is a serious disease; the average patient survives only about five years. It requires much detailed attention and a variety of drugs to help strengthen the heart, to improve excretion of fluids and salt from the kidneys, to control high blood pres-

Pareto Principle

sure and cholesterol and prevent further damage to the heart, and so on. For some patients, a pacemaker may be useful, especially one of the newer pacemakers that have multiple leads to different areas of the heart to help the heart beat at a more effective rate and in a more coordinated manner (what was suggested but not needed for Sophia). But eventually the heart failure progresses to the point where the patient either dies or needs a transplant. In short, heart failure is a serious disease that requires a great deal of specialized attention over time. These patients need a team care approach with one physician orchestrating the work of everyone else on the team. The team can incorporate some "telehealth" or "e-health" strategies here as well. For example, the patient can use a digital scale to weigh himself each morning. The digital scale can automatically send the patient's weight via the Internet to a central office where it can be plotted with an algorithm and can alert the nurse or the physician if the patient's weight is rising. If so, it will prompt a phone call to the patient, perhaps leading to a change in the patient's diuretics and ultimately prevent a trip to the doctor's office, a visit to the emergency room, or even a hospitalization. It is all about integrating telemedicine with good team care.

There is no substitute for having a single physician (or nurse practitioner or other provider) paying attention to the patient and all of his or her problems, but unfortunately it is often not the case. Patients with multiple problems tend to see multiple doctors. Again recall the story of Henry (in chapter 8) who was prescribed twenty-three different medications and saw four different doctors.

I am very proud of the University of Maryland Greenebaum Cancer Center (where I was the director long ago) for its team-based, multidisciplinary approach to care.[4] Revisiting Mr. Ehrmann's lung cancer treatment (see chapter 6), the follow-up is an example of how the team approach works and why it is superior to the usual way cancer care is provided.

After three months of delayed action, Mr. Ehrmann finally had all the required tests done and scheduled a follow-up appointment with a surgeon at a distant tertiary care hospital. When the surgeon's office delayed seeing him for another two weeks, I heard his story later that day, a Wednesday. I called a colleague at the Greenebaum Cancer Center who felt Mr. Ehrmann needed to be seen by a team—a surgeon, radiation oncologist, and medical oncologist—all at one time for a joint plan. They could see him that Friday. After collecting all of his scans and test results, Mr. Ehrmann and his wife drove the four hours to Baltimore, where the threesome examined him. Then, he and his wife went to lunch while the physicians looked at his CT and PET scans and reviewed all of the laboratory studies. When he came back an hour later, they gave him the joint plan: no need for surgery, start with chemotherapy, and then do radiation therapy. He and his wife could stay at the American Cancer Society Hope Lodge for free when they were in town. "OK," he said, "but I am to see that other surgeon on Monday so why don't I go through with that appointment and see what he says." So they did. The Ehrmanns waited three hours until the surgeon could see them. Then he said he had not yet viewed the PET scan so he could not offer a plan of treatment. "Come back for another appointment."

Basically, outside of Mr. Ehrmann's meeting at the Greenebaum Cancer Center, his experience is the typical way most patients get treated for cancer. A patient goes to one doctor and, once he or she is done with his or her recommendation, gets shunted off to the next physician and then the next. The patient may be sent to another physician for a second opinion, but rarely do the doctors actually sit down together and talk through the issues. When a team jointly discusses a patient's situation, jointly listens to the patient's (and the family's) needs, and then jointly offers a plan, you can bet that the plan will be far superior and that there will be no second-guessing later. And as treatment progresses, the team can monitor progress and make course corrections as necessary. The multidisciplinary care coordination approach is not simply better; it is far superior. Accept no substitutes![5]

SUMMARY

Primary care is the linchpin of medical care and health care, but there is a serious shortage of PCPs and it is getting worse. Our perverse insurance system initiated the decline and continuously aggravates the problem such that the current situation leads to a non-sustainable business model for the doctor. Primary care physicians have responded by increasing the number of patients followed, but this means little or no time for good preventive care or care coordination. Any fix must reduce the PCP's load to a reasonable number of patients under care, shift the PCP from being an intervener to an orchestrator, and lead to the PCP's commitment to multidisciplinary, team-based care with full use of adjunct providers. To achieve this goal, and assuming that neither Medicare nor commercial insurance will ever pay adequately for the PCPs' services, the PCPs will need to bill patients and have them pay directly out of pocket, convert to retainer-based practices, or leave independent practice and join organizations that can provide the required arrangements. Personally, I have become an advocate for either direct billing of the patient or the retainer-based model.

$$14$$

Some Final Thoughts on
Cost Management

Misconception: *New technologies increase costs, reduce productivity, and have little beneficial effect on safety or quality care.*

A seventy-three-year-old man needed to have a new heart valve put in to replace a calcified and hardened aortic valve. The patient was brought to the operating room and put to sleep, and the surgery began. The patient was placed on a heart-lung machine, the heart was stopped and opened, and the surgeon announced that he needed a size 25 valve. The scrub nurse says that she has on her tray a size 21, a size 23, and a size 27 but not a size 25. The surgeon knows that the size 27 valve will be too big for the patient's heart, and a size 23 will be too small, leaving the patient's heart unable to pump enough blood through the opening. He is clear that he needs a size 25 for this patient.

An immediate hunt goes on in the storeroom to see if a size 25 valve is available. It is not. After multiple phone calls to the other hospitals in the city that do open-heart surgery, the team learns that one of the hospitals across town does in fact have a size 25 aortic valve available. A nurse is sent out to the front of the hospital, where she grabs a cab to race across town. Unfortunately, it is the morning rush hour, so the going is slow. But she gets across town, and another nurse literally is standing at the hospital's front door with a package holding the size 25 heart valve. The cab heads back across town, the nurse runs up to the operating room, and the valve is inserted into the patient. As it turns out, everything went well with the exception that the patient was on the heart-lung machine for forty-five minutes longer than would have been necessary. From the perspective of the patient's safety and quality of care, the extra time was not a trivial issue. Further, it also meant that that OR was not available on time for the next case.

Had radio frequency identification devices been universally employed in the hospital, the staff would have known before the case began that there was no size 25 valve in the hospital. Why? Because as the equipment, instruments, and materials were brought into the OR, the sensor at the OR door would have recorded each of them. The lack of a size 25 valve would have created an alert long before the patient was even in the operating room.

Putting it all together, there are many reasons why medical care costs are high, but the most important reasons are few: the lack of coordinated care for those with chronic illnesses, personal behaviors that lead to these chronic illnesses, inappropriate or excess use of new technologies, and an organizational inattention to safety. Addressing these causes is where the greatest effort should be placed to start controlling rising medical care costs. It requires a change in the way both commercial and government-sponsored insurance functions. Modifying the malpractice liability system, having an effective electronic medical record, and using eMedicine techniques will also impact both costs and quality. We now know that new technologies, when improperly used, are a big driver of added expenditures, but we also need to realize that new technologies—drugs, devices, imaging—can advance our ability to restore, repair, or replace organs and tissues; to develop entirely new breakthroughs, such as genomics or stem cells; and to devise ways to prevent illnesses from ever occurring, such as with new vaccines. Properly considered, new technologies can be a major factor in reducing medical expenditures.

Throughout this book I have advocated for high-deductible health insurance policies and have been positive about the development of retainer-based primary care practices. Is this advocacy just my opinion, or is there some data to support these contentions? The answer is that the data for the former is pretty good, although not perfect, and for the latter is mostly based on interviews. The RAND Corporation evaluated over 800,000 households from 53 different corporations where 28 offered both a high-deductible policy (HDHP) and a more typical preferred-provider organization (PPO). For those who selected the HDHP option, the total expenditures were 14 percent less than in the PPO option. It was interesting that the savings only occurred if the deductible was $1,000 or more; not if the deductible was less. In many instances, the employer contributed a sum to the person's HSA, and in those cases the savings tended to be less, suggesting it has to be your own money at risk, and it needs to be sufficient (in this case above $1,000) to lead to lower costs. The RAND investigators found some evidence of reduced use of preventive care in the HDHP group. This was interesting because the plans had exclusions for preventive care, meaning that the plan would pay for it, not the individual.[1]

Aetna offers consumer-directed health plans (CDHP), which have three key characteristics: an HSA; a high deductible but with an exclusion for preventive care, including immunizations and an annual examination; and access to certain information tools to aid the patient in decision making. Aetna analyzed their data from 2004 and found that those in a CDHP experienced a lower rise in health expenditures than those in their other PPO-type plans. Unlike RAND, Aetna found greater use of preventive care among these individuals.[2] Aetna refers to a study by Mercer, done in 2005, showing that the cost per employee enrolled in a CDHP was $5,233 compared to $6,095 for those in the more typical PPO plans; like in the RAND study, this was a 14 percent reduction.

These studies indicate that the use of a high deductible will reduce costs substantially, and may not adversely affect use of preventive care (as in the Aetna study). With the health reform legislation, preventive care must be paid by the insurer, so that issue should become moot, provided that the individual is made aware that preventive care is available at no added cost. Of course, it could be argued that those who selected the HDHP may have just been those who were inherently more likely to be cautious in the use of their medical benefits. I disagree. My own transition over a few years as revealed by my stories of the betamethasone prescription, the requested repeat vocal cord examination, the suggestion that I have an annual cardiac stress test and a few others not included have taught me that a high deductible is a strong motivator to ask questions and challenge advice. Another argument against the use of HDHP is that the person with serious chronic illnesses will end up needing to pay more for care and as a result may choose to not get the care really needed. The answer here is to be sure you understand all the costs up front. Most HDHP have dollar limits for your out-of-pocket costs. Check these out up front when you choose your plan.

What about retainer-based primary care? The field is too new for any useful studies to have been done. I therefore have relied on my interviews and experience. The PCPs I talked to who have made the switch are unanimous: they now give much superior care in a very improved setting and, as one put it, "Now I have time to think." And what about the patients? My nonscientific poll of perhaps twenty individuals who have gone through the transition with their physicians all report a superior sense of care and attention. They may not prefer to pay extra, but as one put it, "It is not much more than I pay for my iPhone and data plan, and it is much more important." But no matter how you cut it, that $1,500 or $2,000 is an extra payment for you above and beyond your insurance premiums.

Following are some additional thoughts on cost management in health-care delivery.

HARNESS TECHNOLOGIES TO REDUCE EXPENDITURES

Rather than perceive technologies as exacerbating the cost crisis, it is quite possible to use technology to cut expenditures if properly considered and deployed. It need not be true that new technologies simply increase the total cost of care, as the misconception at the beginning of this chapter suggests. Distance medicine conducted through telemedicine, teleconsults, and e-mails can reduce the need for office visits, the likelihood of going to the emergency room, and unnecessary hospitalizations. These savings all obviously will reduce overall costs, but currently the payment system does not offer reimbursement for telemedicine, teleconsults, and e-mail exchanges. Similarly, there is no reimbursement for tele-diagnostic devices, such as the electronic home scale that reports a patient's daily weight to the physician's office. Reimbursement will be necessary if these valuable and cost-saving techniques are to be widely adopted. Should most care in the future become managed via accountable care organizations or should most primary care physicians opt for retainer-based practices, then it is to the physician's benefit rather than a financial loss to use these technologies. Of course, if we were each responsible for paying up to a set deductible for our own routine care, then we also would pay for the convenience and benefits of e-mail interaction with our physicians.

We can harness technologies also to improve safety and quality and, as a result, reduce expenditures. The EMR can have a major impact on quality and safety. Prescribing drugs via the hospital computer, known as computer physician order *CPOE* entry, can eliminate misinterpreting the doctor's illegible handwriting, prevent prescribing a drug to someone who is allergic to it, avoid adverse drug interactions, and assist the physicians in prescribing the correct dose, number of doses per day, and route of administration. With outpatient prescriptions, e-prescribing offers all of the same advantages as CPOE plus the prescription can be sent instantly to the local pharmacy and the medication is ready by the time the patient arrives to pick it up. In the hospital setting, CPOE sends the prescription to the hospital pharmacy immediately. Because it is already digitized, the pharmacist can check the prescription, the technicians and the various robots can prepare and deliver it to the hospital unit, and the patient can receive it in prompt order.

Other important technologies that can help reduce costs are simulators, robots, and identification devices. Simulation is used for procedure training, practice, and certification. Indeed, simulation, as described in the opening story in chapter 6, will profoundly impact the safety and quality of operative procedures, cardiac catheterization, colonoscopy, and many other procedures and, in turn, drastically affect their associated cost management. Simulation can shorten the time it takes to become proficient, thereby reducing training time and costs.

I have mentioned using robots in the OR (see chapter 4) and in the pharmacy (chapter 6). The pharmacy robots include one that selects drugs by their bar codes or RFID tags, another that prepares the intravenous medications and always draws up the exact amount, and the robot that can deliver the drugs to the patient's unit.

Another technology that can help reduce expenditures is the radiofrequency identification device, along with other identification technologies. Just as Wal-Mart has pioneered the using these tags to manage their inventory, so, too, can hospitals. Consider the actual OR situation described at the beginning of this chapter. RFID and similar technologies can ensure that the OR is properly prepared and ready at the start of each case. They can indicate whether all of the staff—the surgeon, anesthesiologist, scrub nurse, and so on—are available and can pinpoint where the patient is (maybe taken to X-ray or even to the wrong OR). RFID can keep track of medication inventories and all of the other supplies that a hospital needs. In the process it can greatly facilitate just-in-time stocking and keep inventory levels adequate but not excessive. It would have prevented the sorry situation that occurred with the heart surgery patient described at the start of this chapter. While that story was about patient safety and quality, the root cause of the problem was a supply chain management system that could stand improvement.

IMPROVED PATIENT EDUCATION AND INVOLVEMENT
IN DECISION MAKING

Traditionally, a physician told a patient that he or she had a certain problem and what the treatment was. The patient was expected to nod, take the prescription to the pharmacy, and follow directions without asking many questions. This relationship has obviously changed considerably. Doctors are more likely to explain their reasoning, and patients are more likely to ask more questions. But the patient is still at a disadvantage in this discussion because of the information gap between patient and physician. The result is that all too often the discussion is not in-depth and the patient does not feel as if he or she is in a position to challenge the physician's advice, especially in acute or emergent situations. This situation is beginning to change for the patient with a complex, chronic disease such as diabetes, heart failure, rheumatoid arthritis, or lupus. More and more, patients talk to friends with the same illness or search the Internet for, hopefully valid, information. This education is to the patient's benefit, but with physicians having only a short time to interact with each patient, the patient's effort is still not sufficient.

Doctors need to recognize this information imbalance and strive to correct it. Often we leave the doctor's office only to have forgotten some or much of what was discussed because we were anxious during the visit. It is important to have follow-up information once at home. I am familiar with a team that conducts initial evaluations of breast cancer patients, and it prints out the recommendations for the patient after they have had a full discussion and before she leaves the consultation room. The document includes extensive information about her unique situation and the proposed specific approach to treatment. With this printout in hand, the patient and her family can read it when they get home. This simple process leads to better care, a more informed patient, and a big reduction in stress and turmoil. And it means fewer calls to the team for clarifications.

Physicians need to be absolutely certain that the patient understands what is being recommended, why, and what the risks and possible adverse consequences might be for any treatment. Patients need to be insistent and ask questions, without feeling stigmatized for it, until they feel fully informed. Patients also need to be kept updated and then allowed to participate in the decisions about their medical care. This style of communication is a cultural change for the patient and for the doctor, but it is essential to ensure high-quality care at a more reasonable cost. Leveling the information gap will improve quality and reduce expenditures. The patient needs to realize, however, that he or she might have to pay the physician for taking the extra time needed to provide this information exchange. (Unfortunately, many insurers including Medicare do not allow such extra "side" payments to physicians.)

ACADEMIC MEDICAL CENTERS

Many believe that a sure way to improve care quality and reduce costs, yet maintain or enhance the physician-patient relationship, is to create more integrated delivery systems along the lines of Kaiser Permanente or the Cleveland Clinic. These systems reduce the use of unnecessary specialist consults, tests, procedures, and hospitalizations by combining good care coordination and effective disease prevention. They work, in part, because of their patient-centered culture and their use of good electronic medical records. They also use a prospective payment system, or capitation, rather than only a fee-for-service system. They tend to focus on offering quality care and on achieving patient expectations for satisfaction, which combined has led to reduced total expenditures. They also tend to be cognizant of outcome measures, not only for quality and satisfaction but for safety as well.

Academic medical centers, which are a combination of a tertiary teaching hospital, a medical school, and a faculty practice organization, can lead the way in organizing systems of coordinated care for complex, chronic illness. They have the advantages of being a hospital and training physicians all under one roof, with some of the most specialized caregivers and centers for disease-oriented care such as cancer and trauma centers. But The AMCs' faculty physicians do not function as a coordinated group, as they do at Mayo or Marshfield; rather, they are separate groups of specialists—say, cardiologists, pulmonologists, general surgeons, and so on—without an innate sense of total collaboration. AMCs should study their practice structures and change them to accommodate multidisciplinary teams and care coordination. As part of this approach, they need to integrate much more fully the skills and expertise of other health-care providers—nurses, advanced practice nurses, pharmacists, dentists, and more—into the team. Their success would dramatically improve the care of patients with complex, chronic illnesses.

Physicians tend to work alone; indeed, the whole licensing concept is meant to ensure a practitioner is competent to enter independent practice. However, I have argued here for the use of multidisciplinary teams in which, for example, a surgeon, an internist, and a radiation oncologist would treat the patient with cancer. This concept should and must be broadened to include nurses, nurse practitioners, pharmacists, dentists, physical therapists, social workers, and others.

As an intern at Yale New Haven Hospital I quickly learned that the nurses were critical to my ability to care for patients successfully. When I first joined the

National Cancer Institute (NCI), I was fresh out of residency and thought I knew a great deal about drugs. But at the NCI I had the great benefit of working with expert pharmacists and soon learned that not only did they know more about medications than I did, but they were also my great allies in patient care. Similarly, I began to work with a group of dentists interested in oral care of patients with leukemia; once again I learned that they knew much more about oral diagnosis and oral care than I ever would. Pharmacists and dentists became my mentors and collaborators, and together as we cared for patients, we developed some useful care protocols through research, which led to publications in professional journals that have stood the test of time nationally and internationally. The same can be said of my working with nurses, nurse practitioners, and social workers.

The point is that each profession with its different training and culture has positive skills to contribute. AMCs could—and should—emphasize this fact and build training programs to ensure that that coordinated care is learned. As an example, Jay Perman, MD, president of the University of Maryland–Baltimore with its six health and human services schools, conducts a weekly "president's clinic," where he sees his own pediatric gastroenterology patients, many of whom he has cared for for years. He and his nurse practitioner (he has been working with a nurse practitioner for decades) see each patient. Per session they include a student from each of the schools of medicine, nursing, dentistry, pharmacy, social work, and, yes, even law. The students appreciate the experience and quickly learn that there are various points of view and varying approaches, each of which has validity and adds quality to the totality of patient care. As Dr. Perman likes to say and repeated in his inauguration address, paraphrasing an adage from Robert Fulghum's book *All I Really Need to Know I Learned in Kindergarten*, "It is still true, no matter how old you are, when you go out into the world it is best to hold hands and stick together." Developing this cooperative approach is the challenge of medicine, of primary care, and of academic medical centers.

At AMCs, faculty physicians, by definition, have multiple responsibilities for not only patient care but also research and education. They have the potential and the opportunity to make a real difference in the future of health care. They could change the landscape of how care is coordinated and at the same time teach the principles of coordinated care to students and residents from the beginning. The barriers to their success are high, but if the leaders could only agree on how to proceed, improvements promoted by their success would far outweigh the work to overcome the barriers. It would be a real advance for the country and a powerful marketing tool for the academic health centers. I hope they can step up to this challenge.

I have given you an overview of what needs to be done to improve the quality of medical care, which, in turn, will markedly lower its costs. But achieving these new approaches will not come easily. Indeed, it will be a monumental struggle.

BARRIERS TO SUCCESS

What then will be the barriers to success? Certainly the insurance industry has barriers to reform the insurance methodology. The insurance industry will resist the call to pay higher reimbursement for primary care physicians; incentives for behavior modification; increased reimbursements required for team care, care management, and disease management; and compensation for distance medicine, such as the use of e-mail, telemedicine, and teleconsults. The insurance industry wants to reduce its costs today and not its possible costs tomorrow, even if that reduction could be substantial. A critical reason from its perspective is that individuals change insurance carriers on a regular basis. Insurance companies know that their likelihood of keeping an individual on their rolls for more than a few years can be quite low. As a result their incentive is toward short-term, immediate cost reductions as opposed to programs which in and of themselves cost extra money, even though that extra expenditure could lead to an overall major reduction of costs later on. The CareFirst Blue Cross/Blue Shield program described in chapter 12 is predicated on the observation that the company can keep turnover limited.

Medicare, however, does not have the same excuse. It has each of us from age sixty-five until our last breath. It is in Medicare's best financial interest to encourage and support prevention and care coordination systems that work.

Changing the insurance methodology that we have today will also meet with union and employee resistance. The idea of switching from a company-provided health benefit to one in which the employee owns and pays for the policy will be perceived as a loss of a major benefit. Likewise, switching from what is essentially prepaid medical care today to a policy that is fundamentally for catastrophic care combined with a high deductible will also be perceived as losing a major benefit. In addition, many will perceive making premiums higher for those individuals with certain high-risk behaviors, such as smoking or being overweight, as unfair or even "un-American."

The pharmaceutical companies will resist the concept that they must sell drugs in the United States at the same price for which they are sold in other countries. The United States is their cash cow right now, and they will work aggressively to maintain that enviable position. For the same reason, they will lobby actively to prevent further FDA restrictions or regulations on their advertising to the general population since it has succeeded in generating more prescriptions.

Our cultural expectation that we will not be allowed to die without every conceivable medical approach being considered and tried is deeply ingrained both among patients and physicians. Our teaching approach in medical schools and hospital residency programs is a part of the problem. Watch television shows featuring doctors and see how the residents do every possible test to make a diagnosis and then recommend every conceivable approach to treat a patient well after there is any reasonable hope or expectation for a successful outcome. Unfortunately, these shows mirror reality.

In changing our behaviors, we will have to overcome our own personal resistance. Further, our efforts also will be strongly resisted by the fast-food industry, the commodity agriculture industry, the tobacco industry, and many others that have a huge financial stake in our continued behaviors that lead to poor health.

There also will be major barriers to creating the types of care coordination systems that I have envisioned. Doctors will be concerned about losing their autonomy, which has been a basic aspect of the medical profession for decades, indeed, centuries. Hospitals compete with each other and will be hard-pressed to work together unless they are part of a merged hospital system. Academic medical centers, which could and indeed should take the lead in providing and teaching both sound preventive care and coordinated care of chronic illness and the value of interdisciplinary team care, will resist the necessary changes because it is contrary to the way they are culturally and structurally organized. Independent diagnostic centers and surgicenters will be concerned that their business model will be damaged. And all of them will be correct. When the reforms I propose work effectively, they will reduce the use of unnecessary tests, procedures, devices, surgeries, doctor visits, and hospitalizations—all the things that generate revenues for each entity.

Moving to a coordinated care system would decrease dramatically the total expenditures for medical care. This change needs to occur. Somehow we need to find a way to overcome the barriers and create a better health system for all. The result will be much better quality of care, a much more satisfied patient and family, and substantial reductions in expenditures. And we know that it will work because it is working now in many large clinics, in certain specialty care centers, and in some primary care practices today.

─── KEY STEPS IN REDUCING MEDICAL EXPENDITURES

- Incentivize primary care physicians to carefully coordinate the care of those with chronic, complex illnesses, and assist the PCP in becoming an orchestrator rather than an intervener.

- Create incentives for specialists to work together in multidisciplinary care teams—that is, establish a group of physicians of varying specialization along with nurses, nurse practitioners, pharmacists, social workers, and others—for the care of complex diseases.

- Encourage academic medical centers to create effective integrated systems of care and to teach by example the value of interdisciplinary approaches to care.

- Provide incentives for physicians to offer time with their patients, especially for preventive care.

- Motivate all of us to live a healthier lifestyle both with insurance rates based on weight, lifestyle choices (such as smoking), preventive measures (vaccines and screening tests), and with incentives via workplace, retirement or church-based wellness programs.

- Create a national board to examine evidence-based medicine and make the results broadly available to the physician and patient alike on the Web.

- Use nonprofit and nonbiased organizations, such as the ECRI Institute (formerly the Emergency Care Research Institute), to assist in evaluating devices, tests, and procedures.

- Establish a readily accessible comparative database on drug effectiveness and costs.

- Consider care costs in three major categories:
  annual exams and preventive care, including screening and vaccines
  routine but unexpected medical care
  highly expensive and catastrophic care

- Change the insurance policy approach to
  insure the highly expensive and catastrophic illnesses and events with the
  use of a high deductible

expect unexpected care needs to be paid with savings placed into health savings accounts, which must be available to all

make annual and routine preventive care to be paid out of pocket, preferably with tax advantaged dollars such as with HSAs

create the incentives for physicians noted earlier

appoint the patient as the policyholder or owner regardless of who pays what portion

require all individuals to have catastrophic, high-deductible insurance

reimburse, once the high deductible has been reached, for care coordination, multidisciplinary teams, and eMedicine—e-mails, telemedicine, telediagnosis, and e-prescriptions

- Provide government assistance so those who cannot afford catastrophic insurance and preventive care can obtain them.

- Require electronic medical record and medical device vendors to use interoperability standards.

- Allow each individual to have immediate access to their medical record, paper or digital, after every encounter with the medical care system.

- Overhaul medical malpractice liability to encourage explanation, apology, prompt payment for harm, and careful analysis to prevent similar errors in the future.

- Encourage physicians to spend the time necessary to have meaningful conversations with patients and their families regarding end-of-life care options.

- Help physicians appreciate and call upon the expertise of others, such as nurse practitioners.

- Urge physicians not to order those tests, procedures, and specialist consults unless truly required for patient care and only prescribe drugs that are required or known to be efficacious for the specific situation.

In essence, this list outlines a set of *rights and responsibilities* for the patient and the provider. If the system is adjusted so that each has the necessary rights and responsibilities and the incentives to achieve them, the quality of care will rise substantially, our population will be healthier, and the costs will decline considerably.

PART IV
HEALTH-CARE REFORM

In this section I will first address the critical issues confronting the delivery of medical care in America. Next, I will quickly summarize reform recommendations and look at how Americans disagree on the need for change in medical care and its financing (these differences largely drove the separate approaches recommended by the Republicans and by the Democrats). The final legislation largely reflected the opinions of the Democratic majority in Congress, but there is still much to be determined through the writing of policies and regulations. Already affected organizations and conservative politicians have launched aggressive attempts to repeal the law, to modify it, or to have it deemed unconstitutional by the courts. But even assuming no modifications are enforced, this legislation, although greatly expanding coverage, will not likely improve health-care quality or reduce expenditures in a meaningful way. I will, therefore, offer suggestions along with a summary of actions that could correct some of the current critical deficiencies in medical care delivery. Finally, I will recommend to you, the reader, what you personally can do now to improve your health and keep your expenses down.

15

What Reform Looks Like: Differing Views

Misconception: *Health-care reform will offer access to all, or nearly all, while reducing the costs of care.*

To review, the most critical issues confronting American health care are: effectively reducing the costs of medical care or, at a minimum, slowing the rate of cost escalation; creating access to medical care for the uninsured; changing the way we pay for health care; modifying the negative aspects of the current insurance system; assuming a level of responsibility for our individual health; and improving the quality and the safety of the care we receive. While all of these matters need to be addressed, each one has met substantial resistance from entrenched interests. Personally, I believe that addressing the twin issues of quality and costs was and remains the most important starting point along with a nationwide effort to improve disease prevention. We need a health-care delivery system that closely coordinates the care of those individuals who develop complex, chronic illnesses and catastrophic disease or injury. More than anything else, this effort will begin to reduce the cost of medical care, which has risen so high and so rapidly. It will do so by improving quality and safety. To achieve care coordination will require appropriate financial incentives to primary care physicians (and to some specialists) to accept this added responsibility, along with some incentives for health systems to do the same for those with catastrophic injury or disease. By doing so, the quality of care will rise dramatically.

The health-care reform legislation will go a long way to providing universal coverage but likely will not move us far enough toward proper stewardship of our health-care resources. We need to pay close attention to quality, efficiency, safety, and cost effectiveness.[1] Concurrently, we need to address wellness and prevention.

Workplace wellness programs have been proven to reduce cost escalation, improve health, and enhance worker productivity. Critical to effective wellness programs is the assumption of personal responsibility for a healthier lifestyle—for instance, eating better, losing weight, stopping smoking, and taking blood pressure or high cholesterol medications—in return not only for better health but also for a meaningful economic reward. Allowing insurers to incentivize patients toward wellness with premium reductions is another critical approach to disease prevention. Incentivizing PCPs to give good preventive care and guidance will be important as well.

While the government's reform efforts will be significant, insurers, industry, providers, and all of us can do a great deal now. Insurers can create incentives for care coordination and prevention, industry can develop wellness programs, providers can attend to care coordination and prevention, and all of us can take responsibility for maintaining our own health. The federal and state governments' role is to allow these incentives to occur while creating the governing policies for everyone to follow. These steps alone would improve the quality of care monumentally and lower the total costs of health care.

Various care models have been discussed in this volume. Among them was the CareFirst Blue Cross/Blue Shield plan to increase payments and return a portion of the total savings to the PCPs for chronic illness care coordination and preventive care of their presumably fewer patients (see chapter 12). Another model is that of the Erickson Retirement Communities, where using a Medicare Advantage capitated program the PCPs limit their practices to about four hundred residents each, address geriatric care needs, offer care coordination, visit hospitalized patients, and make extensive use of an electronic medical record (see chapter 8). They also offer wellness programs for the residents along with intellectual stimulation and exercise programs. Yet another model is the Healthy Howard program, which combines both rights and responsibilities for those without health insurance (see chapter 3). The individual may purchase, at a minimal fee, unlimited access to a primary care physician with care coordination and a pharmacy benefits manager to assist with prescriptions. The individual is expected to work with a health coach and accept milestones toward healthier living.

A long-standing approach is the staff model health maintenance organization such as that of Kaiser Permanente. In its complete form, the individual's insurance premium covers all care within Kaiser from the PCP to the specialist to outpatient procedures to hospitalization at a Kaiser hospital. In effect, and key to the HMO's success, all care is bundled so that the entire organization is accountable for the patient's needs. It is in the best interests of the HMO to deliver good preventive care and careful coordination for chronic illnesses because it improves participants' health and reduces costs. Not many true HMOs exist, although those individuals who participate in them generally give them high marks. A variant is the large clinic model—for example, the Mayo, Cleveland, Geisinger, and Dean Clinics—that incorporates primary care and specialist physicians under a single roof, with or with out an owned hospital. Having many, but not necessarily all or even most, patients in a capitated plan drives the clinic staff to treat everyone as though they had prepaid care.

Some PCPs have converted to retainer-based practices. Having fewer patients, spending more time per patient encounter, and paying attention to prevention and chronic illness care coordination markedly improve patient care and satisfaction for both the patients and the doctors.

In all of these programs or models, the basic concept is to offer higher quality medical care, preventive care, and wellness encouragement with the anticipation that costs will be controlled as well as patients' health enhanced. Most pair some level of rights with some expectations of responsibility for the doctor, the hospital, and the patient. In each model, the payment system has been modified from the usual pay-per-visit or procedure model, but not all systems have completely bundled services. For example, Erickson Retirement Communities' residents still see specialists not employed on campus, and many Kaiser HMO participants cannot find a Kaiser-owned hospital nearby.

What is becoming clear, however, is the importance of combining rights (for example, access and care for the individual and increased payments and incentives for the physician or hospital) with responsibilities (healthy living and following a care plan by the individual and coordinating chronic care and offering preventive care by the physician) while at the same time strengthening the direct professional connection between the patient and the primary care provider. In workplace wellness programs the concept is similar as the individual gets an incentive (right) in return for improving current adverse behaviors (responsibility). When properly designed, incentives both enhance quality and reduce costs.

Let's look more at this issue of responsibility.

PERSONAL RESPONSIBILITY VERSUS ACCESS FOR ALL

In 2007 M. G. Bloche made an interesting case for why we should no longer look to the federal government for all-encompassing health care and why we should expect and accept to take more responsibility for our own health care and its financing into the future.[2] He wrote:

> In the summer of 1793, as Prussian and Hapsburg armies closed in on Paris, French leaders issued an unprecedented decree, ordering all unmarried men 18 to 25 years of age to take up arms, married men to make arms, women to sew tents and uniforms, and old men to "excite the courage of the warriors" and "preach the hatred of kings." France thereby transformed warfare from the business of professionals to the work of a whole nation. Historian and legal scholar Philip Bobbitt suggests that we owe our national social-insurance systems to this reinvention of war.

Bloche observes that following this trend to drafted armies, in 1870 Germany linked conscription to the creation of social welfare nets including medical care. This was followed after World War I with further movement in many European countries toward systems of national health insurance. Then came World War II and "for a generation or more, an ethos of reciprocal sacrifice and social obligation lingered in the United States. This ethos helped to create Medicare and Medicaid, enacted in 1965 over opposition from an array of interests." But he argues that now "no longer do most Americans expect to be called on to make the ultimate sacrifice for their country, and no longer do they look to government to provide for their well-being in exchange for their readiness to do so." Although the former is now true, I am not certain that the latter is the shared belief of most or even many Americans. Nevertheless, he suggests that Americans are less inclined to believe that health care is a right. Rather, there is a growing consensus, he believes, that everyone has the obligation to have medical insurance and also to take greater responsibility for their health and wellness. He suggests that "high-deductible coverage, financial rewards for regular workouts and weight control, and penalties (such as premium surcharges) for failure to comply with treatment" are outgrowths of this ethos: "The new compact is likely to start with an enhanced sense of individual obligation—to eat sensibly, exercise regularly, avoid smoking, and otherwise care for ourselves." He predicts that individual obligations with regard to health promotion and disease prevention will increase, as will an obligation to be insured while government will be expected to offer a safety net. He notes that the presidential candidates in the primary and general elections in 2008 did not push for a single government payer system akin to some European countries. He suggests that an approach that balances rights with responsibilities "responds to the anxieties of working Americans, who accept that they must, in the main, depend on themselves. It supplies a safety net when self-reliance falters because of large economic and social forces. And it shields the poor from the degrading, life-endangering consequences of going without basic care because they cannot pay for it. It calls on all of us, though, to take greater personal responsibility for our health, by caring for our bodies and buying insurance."

Certainly not all would or do agree with Bloche's analysis toward an ethic that calls on us to take care of ourselves and to accept responsibility for our own health. It sounds reasonable, but our government leaders in the health reform legislation have not adopted that philosophy. Rather, their philosophy has been one of arranging care coverage for all or nearly all using current methods of insurance from commercial or government sources with some modifications for preexisting conditions and other real problems with current insurance. Their model has limited cost management approaches other than further restrictions on price, but that philosophy has borne no value over the past few decades. Further, it pays inadequate attention to care quality or patient safety.

THE FUNDAMENTAL DIFFERENCES BETWEEN REPUBLICANS AND DEMOCRATS

It is instructive to look at how Americans have perceived the needs of health-care reform. The Kaiser Family Foundation did a survey in the summer of 2007, well before the presidential primaries pushed the issue into the national consciousness, and well before the financial meltdown in the fall of 2008. It found that those who consider themselves Republicans hold quite different views from those who label themselves as Democrats.[3] Jonathan Oberlander, in an article for the *New England Journal of Medicine*, highlighted these differences and then contrasted them with what the presidential candidates were proposing.[4] Not surprising, the candidates generally mirrored their basic constituents in their proposals.

In that Kaiser poll, 67 percent of Democrats but only 35 percent of Republicans opted for a proposal for a "new health care plan that would make a major effort to provide insurance to all or nearly all of the uninsured and would involve a substantial increase in spending." Contrast this finding with the 55 percent of Republicans compared to 24 percent of Democrats who instead favored either a "new health plan that is more limited . . . and would involve less spending" or a "health plan that would keep things basically as they are." Independents straddled the two groups in their views. Another way to look at this information is that Democrats clearly tended toward universal insurance coverage whereas Republicans were split among the three possible options offered in the survey. These views held up in repeated surveys through the presidential election, the economic downturn of 2008–2009, and the congressional debates on health-care reform.

Given that Democratic and Republican voters had contrasting views on health care reform, not surprisingly the issue played out differently in the parties' presidential primaries. The leading Democratic candidates all released comprehensive, detailed plans that were remarkably similar. Most aimed to cover all or nearly all uninsured Americans, to build on the current mixed system of private and public insurance, and to avoid making any changes that would unsettle people who are currently insured. As to the Republicans, they tended as a group to focus more on market reforms that would drive down the price of insurance, offer some reform of the malpractice process, and give a nod toward preventive health care.

By October 2008, right before the election, 75 percent of Democrats and 61 percent of independents thought that "given the economic challenges facing the country it is more important than ever to take on health care reform" compared to only 42 percent of Republicans where the alternative answer was "we cannot take on health care reform right now." About half of all respondents, Republican or Democrat, thought that the first priority should be "making health care and health insurance more affordable," whereas 35 percent of Democrats, but only 9 percent of Republicans, selected "expanding health insurance coverage for the uninsured" as their top choice. Members of both parties believed that reducing health-care costs would have a positive impact on the overall economy. To get there, Democrats, by 61 percent compared to 23 percent of the Republicans, believed more federal regulation would be helpful; whereas Republicans, by 67 percent compared to 31 percent of the Democrats, recommended competition in the marketplace as the way to reduce costs. Independents were about evenly split between regulation and competition.[5]

So it is clear that differing views on the issues correlate to one's party affiliation to a large degree. It is not surprising that the political leaders of both parties presented widely divergent approaches to health-care reform.

By late 2009, with the debate raging in Congress and the airways and with multiple town hall meetings over the summer giving substantial push back, the numbers in the Kaiser Family Foundation polls had begun to change. The gulf between Democrats and Republicans had become wider than ever. In this and other polls, it was evident that a majority of Americans had come to oppose reform as it was being developed. The December poll showed only 35 percent of Americans felt they would be better off if the reform legislation passed and 31 percent (up from 12 percent eight months earlier) believed the country would be worse off with the legislation.[6] Concerns arose that the reforms would increase, not decrease, the cost of medical care; lead to increased taxes; not improve care quality and could even lessen it; and would expand the national deficit. Within Congress, there was certainly not bipartisan support for reform, and support seemed to be waning into the late winter as a vote approached. The February 2010 nationally televised debate on reform did little to suggest compromise was possible. The final Kaiser poll before the vote in Congress showed 46 percent backed and 42 percent opposed the bill, with 12 percent undecided.[7] In the end, the legislation passed with a narrow majority vote and no Republican backing.

A few observations are fairly obvious. We really do have a crisis in American health care today. It is much too expensive, it is not available to all, and it is not up to the standards of quality that it could or should be, especially given our knowledge and abilities already in place. We have seen that costs are high and rising rapidly; business, government, and individuals simply cannot afford the current costs much less the predictions for even higher costs in the future. The lack of access means that all too many Americans have poor or no care and as a result have developed diseases that could have been controlled at an earlier stage. They have higher death rates and shorter life spans. The key to successful reform lies in improving quality through the coordination and level of care while reducing costs for patients, employers, and government and creating funds to insure those who are less fortunate.

Politicians also recognize, overtly or subconsciously, that decreasing spending for health care, which represents a huge portion of our economy, will mean more job losses during a time of recession. They are loath to be labeled "job destroyers" even though they publicly rail against the high cost of care.

PROPOSALS FOR REFORM

In *Critical: What We Can Do about the Health-Care Crisis*, published shortly before the 2008 presidential election, Senator Tom Daschle, Scott S. Greenberger, and Jeanne M. Lambrew outlined what they believed the Democratic plan for health care should be.[8] One key element was the creation of a Federal Health Board (see chapter 6) charged with "recommending coverage of those drugs and procedures backed by solid evidence." This concept is not new; it was part of the plan then First Lady Hillary Clinton developed in the early 1990s. It would exert influence by ranking services and therapies by their impact on health and cost. The expectation would be for government programs that pay for or provide health care, such as Medicare, Medicaid, Defense Department and Veterans Health Administration, to follow the Federal Health Board's lead; and presumably the private insurers—Blue Cross/Blue Shield, UnitedHealthcare, Aetna, and so on—would follow suit. Daschle's proposed Federal Health Board would be a public-private organization somewhat akin to the Federal Reserve, but designed to monitor and assist the country's health-care system. The president would appoint its governors, who would have to be confirmed by the Senate. Each governor would have well-recognized expertise in health policy, clinical medicine, or both and would serve a ten-year term. The board would have the weighty responsibility of determining what procedures, practices, drugs, devices, and so forth, would be included in the various federal insurance plans and presumably by the Federal Employee Health Benefits Plan (FEHBP), which covers many federal employees, including Congress. Daschle also recommended that FEHBP, a program that offers a menu of private insurance plans, be available to everyone. During the general election, then Senator Obama repeatedly suggested that everyone should be able to access the same plan offered to members of Congress.

Many providers, especially physicians and hospitals along with pharmaceutical and medical device firms through their respective lobbying agents, argued against this proposed National Health Board on the grounds that no group of experts, no matter their good intentions, can or should decide what is right for everyone's medical care. The "average patient" is not necessarily the same as the current patient in the doctor's office. Many will say making these decisions, in effect, is rationing. Providers will argue that they and they alone are best equipped to make these decisions for each individual patient, especially since they know the patient's circumstances. In the final legislation the Daschle concept of a board was not included, but an institute to conduct comparative effectiveness research was funded, superseding that the one created earlier through the stimulus bill (American Recovery and Reinvestment Act of 2008). This institute's board of governors can make recommendations as to findings, but these cannot be construed as mandates, guidelines, or recommendations for payments, coverage, or treatment and cannot be used to deny coverage.

The important issue, to me, is to have good-quality evaluations of current and proposed medical treatments or diagnostic approaches that can guide the practitioner to offer his or her patient the best available management. Hopefully the new institute will prove helpful in understanding what works and what does not, and making that information generally available in a transparent, widely distributed fashion. Doing good comparative effectiveness research will potentially help all of us to either get the treatment we need or to avoid one that does not work. Here is a story about an individual who was offered a therapeutic procedure commonly preformed at the time, but which was later shown in a well done randomized controlled trial to be no better than conventional non-surgical management.

Charlie Phillips was repairing his elevated deck when he fell, hurting his back. When it did not improve in a few days, he visited an orthopedist who offered to insert a cement material into the space where his brittle vertebral bone had been compressed and crushed. Charlie was not prepared to undergo surgery and declined, but six months later, after physical therapy and other conservative measures had not worked, he returned to the orthopedist. "Let's do it," he said. But the physician responded that unfortunately the procedure was only appropriate if done at the onset of the problem. When Charlie told me about his situation, he was frustrated that his initial delay meant he could not pursue the surgical option. As it turns out, though, he was lucky in a strange sort of way. Just a few weeks later, a study reported that the procedure, when compared to placebo surgery, was of no added benefit. Restated, patients who underwent the sham operation had as much improvement as did those who had the actual procedure.[9] This corrective surgery had become very widely used, but now the evidence suggests that it should be used only in some limited circumstances. With this evidence now in, I am pleased that my friend did not undergo needless surgery, although I empathize that he still has much discomfort.

This type of information, based on sound scientific study, is what medical practitioners need. Sometimes it will run counter to what a drug or device manufacturer wants or counter to long-held physician practice patterns. But we still need the information because, per the old maxim, "the truth will set you free." Sometimes, however, the truth will be a bitter pill for someone or some company to have to swallow.

CHANGE, SLOWLY BUT SURELY

We have a system in America that, for all of its faults, has some stability. There are those people on the left and the right who would love dearly to impose major change.

They feel strongly and are adamant in their advocacy, often citing, for example, the systems in other industrialized countries that offer access to all. But as Dr. Atul Gawande has pointed out in the *New Yorker*, those countries with universal health care each got to their current situation from widely different conditions, generally as an aftermath of World War II.[10] The British had to construct a system during the war to address the needs not only of its soldiers and sailors but also those of Britons who were injured or displaced from bombed cities. Expected to be a temporary measure, it became well regarded and was basically continued after the war. France did not have a national health-care system during the war, but it had a system of payroll taxes for various insurance needs. So France built on it and today still uses payroll tax–financed insurance for all, mostly through local, not-for-profit insurers. Switzerland, which avoided the ravages of war, had a system of private commercial health insurance. It built on that system, required everyone to purchase insurance, and set a limit of about 10 percent of earnings as a maximum payment. Each of these systems has worked well, and the populace in each country is generally satisfied. The key point here is that each country built on its own current systems and traditions and did not move to a major new system all of a sudden as the result of government fiat.

Misconception: *Health-care reform will fundamentally improve how we receive care going forward.*

What actually happened? As of this writing (summer of 2011), many people are concerned that the congressionally passed reforms will increase the cost of medical care, will lead to increased taxes, will not improve care quality, and will expand the national deficit. (See for example the various Kaiser Family Foundation health polls referred to at the end of this chapter.) But it will give insurance coverage to an additional 30 plus million Americans now living without insurance, including those people with preexisting conditions. It also extends the time a child can remain on his or her parents' policy, eliminates exclusions for preexisting conditions, and eliminates lifetime caps on benefits. Unfortunately, progress on the difficult-to-achieve costs and quality agenda were marginal at best, as were the goals of improved prevention and public health, whereas the populist goal of expanding coverage will be largely achieved in the coming years. To be fair, there are many pilot programs related to cost and quality embedded in the bill, and some of these may well bear value in the years to come. But to our collective detriment, this imbalance of coverage improvement with limited cost management and quality enhancements will only exacerbate the cost crisis and expand taxes. It will not drive the quality improvements that are desperately needed for everyone, rich or poor, insured or uninsured, healthy or chronically ill.

Rather abruptly, Congress has now begun to address its budget deficit issues and the mounting national debt. During this process, Congressman Paul Ryan proposed a bill that would change Medicare to a voucher system. The Republican-dominated House of Representatives passed the proposal, but it promptly died in the Senate. In June 2011, Senator Joseph Lieberman and Senator Thomas Coburn put forward a bipartisan proposal for Medicare reform. It also received lukewarm responses at best, but the senators point out that Medicare is our largest entitlement and that it needs to be addressed before it becomes the straw that breaks the camel's back, meaning that the expenditures of Medicare are continuing to rise at a time when there is little enthusiasm for increasing taxes to cover the costs.

What is the American people's opinion on the health reform bill as of today? The Kaiser Family Foundation tracking poll in August 2011 shows that 44 percent have an unfavorable opinion of the law, 39 percent a favorable opinion, and 17 percent have no view. These are numbers largely unchanged throughout the monthly polls during 2011. Among Democrats, support has slipped from close to 70 percent to now 60 percent; Republicans are up some, but only to 24 percent; and independents are fairly steady at 33 percent. In other data, 19 percent of those who *have* insurance said they had trouble paying their medical bills, and 20+ percent indicated they had skipped doctor visits, not purchased prescription medications, or used home remedies instead of seeing a physician. Among the uninsured, about one half were not aware of the coming benefits to them of the reform legislation, such as expansion of the Medicaid program.[11]

Following is a summary of some of the key elements of the Patient Protection and Affordable Health Care Act.[12] It is a long and complicated bill, so many but certainly not all of its elements are included here. As these steps move into place over the coming years, what else needs to be done? I will offer my suggestions in the next chapter.

─── AFFORDABLE HEALTH CARE FOR AMERICA ACT (PASSED MARCH 21, 2010): SUMMARY OF KEY ELEMENTS

COVERAGE

- Would expand coverage to 32 million Americans who are currently uninsured, bringing total coverage to about 94 percent of Americans.

- Will augment Medicaid for the poor, creating exchanges for commercial insurance for individual purchase, establishing subsidies for those of lesser means, and requiring commercial insurers to accept all individuals regardless of preexisting conditions. Concurrently, all must agree to purchase insurance, with or without government subsidy assistance, and companies that employ more than 50 individuals have certain requirements to meet or be fined. Businesses with fewer than 25 employees and an average wage of less than $50,000 will be eligible for tax credits.

MEDICAID

- Expands to include all non-elderly Americans with income below 133 percent of the federal poverty level (FPL), which is $22,050 for a family of four; thus, the expansion covers a family of four making less than $29,327.
- Makes the federal government pay all the costs for newly eligible individuals through 2016 (usually states pay about half of the Medicaid costs).
- Increases payments to primary care physicians to levels equivalent to Medicare reimbursements beginning in 2013.

COMMERCIAL INSURANCE

HEALTH INSURANCE EXCHANGES

- Conceptually, the exchanges will leverage group purchasing power, which is currently available only to large employers.
- Exchanges will begin in each state in 2014.
- The uninsured and self-employed not eligible for Medicaid will be able to purchase insurance through state-based exchanges, with subsidies available to individuals and families with income between the 133 percent and 400 percent of the FPL (for a family of four, that would be between $29,327 and $88,200).
- Separate exchanges will be created for small businesses to purchase coverage effective 2014.
- Funding will be available to states to establish exchanges within one year of enactment and until January 1, 2015.
- Illegal immigrants will not be allowed to buy health insurance in the exchanges, even if they pay completely with their own money.

SUBSIDIES

- Individuals and families making 100–400 percent of the FPL who want to purchase their own health insurance on an exchange are eligible for subsidies. They cannot be eligible for Medicare or Medicaid and cannot be covered by an employer. Eligible buyers receive premium credits, and there is a cap for how much they have to contribute to their premiums on a sliding scale.

INDIVIDUAL MANDATE

- In 2014, everyone must purchase health insurance or face a $695 annual fine. There are some exceptions for low-income people.

EMPLOYER REQUIREMENTS

- Employers with more than 50 employees must provide health insurance or pay a fine of $2,000 per worker each year if any worker receives federal subsidies to purchase health insurance.

COMMERCIAL INSURANCE REQUIREMENTS

- Six months after enactment, insurance companies may no longer deny children coverage based on a preexisting condition.
- Companies may no longer impose lifetime limits on coverage or drop individuals who develop illnesses while covered ("rescission").
- Starting in 2014, insurance companies may no longer deny coverage to anyone with preexisting conditions.
- Begun in 2010, young adults may stay on their parents' insurance plans until age twenty-six.
- Certain rules implemented regarding coverage for preventive health care, including elimination of co-pays.

MEDICARE PART A AND B

- Provides physician reimbursement for annual wellness visits, and eliminates co-pays for preventive benefits including mammography and colonoscopy beginning in 2011. No deductibles or co-pays for wellness or preventive services.
- Increases reimbursement to primary care physicians.
- Encourages a change in the payment system from a fee for visit or procedure to a value-based reimbursement.
- Encourages, beginning in 2012, the creation of accountable care organizations (ACOs), or integrated health systems, by incentivizing physicians to join together to improve care coordination, reduce hospitalizations, increase quality, and help to prevent illness.
- Allows physicians to keep a portion of the savings developed.

- Begins to create bundled payments in 2013 among physicians and hospitals for episodes of care with savings shared between Medicare and the providers.

MEDICARE ADVANTAGE PLANS

- Medicare currently pays commercial insurers about $1,000 more per individual than with original Medicare, but this amount will be slowly reduced.

MEDICARE PART D

- This effort closes the Medicare prescription drug "doughnut hole" by 2020, but seniors who reached the doughnut hole by 2010 received a $250 rebate. The current doughnut hole is between $2,700 and $6,154 in drug expenses per year, meaning that the individual must pay the full costs of prescription medications after the first $2,700 has been spent and until $6,154 has been incurred. The hole is closed by a combination of increased benefits and reduced prices by pharmaceutical firms for brand-name medications.
- Beginning in 2011, seniors in the gap will receive a pharmaceutical manufacturers' 50 percent discount on brand-name drugs, rising to 75 percent on both brand-name and generic drugs by 2020.

TOTAL COST TO FEDERAL GOVERNMENT BASED ON CONGRESSIONAL BUDGET OFFICE ANALYSIS

- $940 billion over ten years (additional costs to states for their share of Medicaid expansion).
- Would reduce the deficit by $143 billion over the first ten years.

PAYING FOR REFORM

- New revenues (taxes)

  Medicare payroll tax on investment income: starting in 2012, the Medicare payroll tax will be expanded to include unearned income with a 3.8 percent tax on investment income for families with an adjusted gross income of more than $250,000 per year or an individual with more than $200,000 per year.

  Excise tax: beginning in 2018, insurance companies will pay a 40 percent excise tax on so-called Cadillac, high-end insurance plans worth more than $27,500 for families and $10,200 for individuals. Dental and vision plans are exempt.

Looks good now - but wait for inflation to catch up!

Tanning tax: 10 percent excise tax will be imposed on indoor tanning services.

- Cost reductions for Medicare: $500 billion in next decade

    A reduction in the funding of Medicare Advantage payments by about 14 percent to equal those of fee-for-service Medicare. Current Advantage plans' payment rates will be frozen and then slowly reduced in coming years. Those companies that offer Advantage plans may choose to cut back on benefits currently in excess of those mandated by Medicare.

    A reduction in physician reimbursement of 21 percent. (Very likely this will be eliminated by Congress. It has been a political football for years and appears that it will continue to be so.)

    The creation of an independent Medicare Payment Advisory Board that will make recommendations for saving money.

16

Recommendations for Reform: Aligning Rights with Responsibilities

Misconception: *Health care is or should be a right, not a privilege and not a responsibility.* As we saw in chapter 7, Safeway has made wellness programs available to all of its 30,000 nonunionized personnel. Its program is based on two insights: 70 percent of all medical costs result from adverse behaviors, such as smoking, overeating, and lack of exercise; and 74 percent of all costs are related to four chronic illnesses—cardiovascular, cancer, diabetes, and obesity—and that are, for the most part, preventable with behavior modifications. The program's concept is that if a person agrees to live a healthy lifestyle, then his or her share of the health insurance premiums decreases substantially. Safeway gives classes and counseling in smoking cessation, weight reduction, stress management, and nutrition at no charge.

As of 2010 Safeway had held total all-inclusive per-employee health-care costs at 2005 levels, whereas most other large American companies have seen a cumulative increase of about 50 percent over the same time period. Safeway points out that had the company not actually expanded benefits, its costs would have fallen by 5 percent from 2005 to 2009. In addition it has reported workers are satisfied with the program and have presumed better health, less absenteeism, and improved productivity. Concurrently, the staff is benefiting from lower insurance premiums. Not all of the cost management resulted from financial incentives; indeed, those only began in 2008. Safeway also gives its staff access to a 24/7 nurse hotline, free health screenings, free or discounted gym memberships, and subsidies for weight control programs, and it actively pushes for the use of generic drugs. More staff members have brought their blood pressure, cholesterol, or both under control, and, according to a company spokesman, the rate of obesity, although still too high, has fallen to well below the national average.

Questions have been raised as to how much Safeway's results were due to incentives[1] and others point out that behavioral economics can be used to best design incentive systems.[2] But add the Safeway program to the results of other companies' plans, and it is clear that wellness programs work. Financial incentives add to their value by encouraging workers to commit and stick to the system, and taking responsibility for their own health. Once again, it is all about rights and responsibilities linked together.

Missing from many discussions of health-care reform is this needed balance of responsibilities paired with rights. The two are, or at least should be, linked at every level. The Safeway example of linking rights and responsibilities achieved an excellent outcome. So, too, has the Healthy Howard approach by providing patients access to care and expecting them to participate in boosting their well-being (see chapter 3).

To recap, we have explored four elements that need to be included in any meaningful program of health-care reform. Addressing only one or two will compound the current problems stemming from the other factors. First, to move from our current medical care system to a health-care system, we must address prevention, wellness, and health promotion, largely through paying attention to and modifying our own behaviors and by recognizing the importance of public health measures such as vaccines, safe food, and sanitation. Second, we need to bring down the costs of expensive medical care. Third, we need to organize medical care so that those with complex, chronic illnesses receive quality and safe treatment and support in a well-coordinated system. And, fourth, we need to find a way to offer excellent health care to all regardless of their ability to pay, the status of their health, or their social status provided that they in return take responsibility for their own personal health-care behaviors. Indeed, personal responsibility needs to become part of the equation for all of us; we should not have these rights without accepting our commensurate responsibility. The same stipulation goes for providers, insurers, and the government, which also must balance their rights and responsibilities.

So what needs to be done next? How can competing and differing approaches— those focused on providing universal access versus those committed to quality improvement, those who believe in a government-organized and mandated system versus those committed to a marketplace system with enhanced competition—lead to a grand compromise? Following a brief review is a proposal.

REVIEW

It is important to fully appreciate that most disease is caused over time by our own poor choices concerning weight, nutrition, stress, exercise, smoking, dental hygiene, seat belts and driving, and sex. Moreover, many do not obtain available immunizations and either do not have screening tests (blood pressure, cholesterol, cancer) or else do not respond to their findings. Addressing these behaviors—as difficult as some (such as obesity and smoking) will be—is the real key to improved health and reduced expenditures. Having access to insurance and to physician and hospital care is definitely important but only if we all make real and concerted efforts at using preventive medicine.

The federal and state governments need to make behavior modification an integral aspect of health care and health-care reform. We should discourage the use of processed foods in favor of whole grains, fresh vegetables, and plenty of fruit and discourage sugared foods such as sodas. This focus will mean a marked change for programs in the Department of Agriculture and a recognition that the food pyramid cannot be adjusted for the needs of one farm group, industry, or another. Restaurants and stores that are purveyors of prepared foods must be required to display the ingredients, calories, and fat, carbohydrate, and sodium content of their meals. We also need to be more aggressive about stopping smoking and preventing the habit from forming. Those who are already addicted need help in withdrawing from nicotine.

These topics are not usually talked about, and many politicians will have difficulty entering this arena, but it is essential. If we do not change our behaviors and focus on prevention, we are doomed to have an unhealthy population with increasing rates of complex, chronic lifelong diseases, such as diabetes with serious complications, heart failure, cancer and chronic lung disease, as well as continued high medical care costs. Concurrently, our public health agencies, including the Centers for Disease Control and local health departments, need to be strengthened. The overlapping authorities and responsibilities of the Food and Drug Administration and the Department of Agriculture need to be streamlined with clear accountability for the health of the populace. As noted earlier, I commend First Lady Michelle Obama's encouraging Americans, especially children, to adopt healthier diets. The recent Department of Agriculture's focus on educating Americans to eat more nutritious foods with less sodium and fat and a greater intake of fresh fish is also commendable.

Just to be clear, I definitely do not advocate that the government should impose "lifestyles." Rather, the government should find appealing ways to "nudge" us in the right direction by educating us and creating policies such as financial incentives that assist (not insist) us to reach the goal of healthier living.[3] But we must preserve our right to smoke, to eat poorly, or to be overweight if that is our desire. For those of us who do so insist, however, others should not be responsible for shouldering a substantial part of our medical care costs because of our decisions. We need to be personally responsible for ourselves and not expect or assume that "big brother" in the form of government, taxpayers, or neighbors will help us later. That said, it is important for the government to protect us without taking away others' rights or allowing the costs of others' choices to be transferred to all of us.

Misconception: *The only health-care reform that matters is what the federal government implements; providers and employers can do little.*

American industry has demonstrated with workplace wellness programs that health can be improved while holding down insurance cost escalation. Key elements to their success are appropriate incentives to encourage responsible behavior. These programs need to be extended and replicated across the country, in private industry, on retirement campuses, in church or community-based settings, and in government organizations. It is not appropriate to insist that everyone's premiums should be the same because they live in the same political subdivision; instead, it would be better to insist that those who accept responsibility for a healthy lifestyle should share the same premiums. (To be clear, I am not advocating for "lifestyle police." We should have the right to live as we choose, but those individuals who attempt to live a healthy lifestyle should be rewarded with an opportunity for lower insurance premiums.) Businesses should be allowed to maximize their incentives as they deem appropriate. For example, wellness programs should be able to give an incentive for not smoking against the cost of company-sponsored insurance well above the current federal limit. The ACA will allow this.

Misconception: *If waste in medical care is eliminated or at least markedly curtailed, there will not be a need to limit what insurance covers.*

Unfortunately, there is plenty of waste in today's medical care. Most of it results from poor or inadequate care coordination of patients with chronic illnesses. Henry's story in chapter 8 is a good example. To combat this sort of waste, poor care, low quality, and inadequate safety in today's medical care setting, care must become patient centric, thoroughly coordinated, and focused on prevention. With these changes, waste will drop dramatically.

Other important, direct steps to reduce the costs of care are improving the quality of care and enhancing its safety. The key issue here is to create incentives for PCPs to coordinate care and for disease-oriented teams of providers to deliver complex care in a well-coordinated manner. Coordination of care can be handled by primary care physicians, specialty physicians, or nurse practitioners, or by strengthening incentives, large group practices or multidisciplinary care teams can be developed and organized around the concept of chronic care coordination. Once again, incentives must be created in return for the provider accepting responsibility for managing care effectively and efficiently. Along with wellness management, these programs will vastly help improve our medical and health-care systems while concurrently reducing the total costs of care.

In addition, medical students must be incentivized to become primary care providers, and providers must be reimbursed for spending time with patients for prevention education. Incentives can come from the insurers, from government in the form of Medicare rate adjustments, or from patients who buy into retainer-based practices.

Additional changes to reduce costs would include forcing drug firms to sell their drugs in America at the same price that they do in other countries. The malpractice system must be altered so that it actually compensates the patient promptly while helping to prevent similar mistakes in the future. Physicians and other providers must be held accountable, probably with negative financial incentives, if they do not maintain accepted standards such as hand washing; following protocols for procedures, such as catheter insertion; or observing principles of evidenced-based care. The excessive paperwork involved for physicians and hospitals billing insurance companies must end. It would eliminate most of the armies of people who ensure compliance with the myriad barriers insurers put in place. Concurrently, significantly reducing the number and burden of well-meaning but often unnecessary regulations and mandates placed on providers is needed. In short, it would allow nurses, physicians, pharmacists, and others to spend more time, not less time, with their patients. These and other steps that have been detailed earlier will have a major impact on reducing costs, improving care, and boosting the morale and spirits of those dedicated to caring for patients.

As previously noted, the United States is the only country in the developed world that does not ensure basic medical care for all of its citizens. Despite major expansion over the past decade of government-funded coverage, especially for children, the number of uninsured has risen to some 47 million Americans. Many others are underinsured, and an increasing number state that they have problems paying for their medical care, owe money, or have been confronted by collection agencies. The reform legislation greatly expands Medicaid, adding some 32 million to the rolls over time. Some states might not be able to afford this added coverage after the initial federal subsidies end, and some states have contested the approach. Equally important, Medicaid pays providers poorly, so it is unclear whether physicians will flock to care for these newly covered individuals.

The ranks of the uninsured are not homogenous. Some are uninsured because they truly cannot afford to pay for coverage or their employers do not offer health insurance. Others, often young and healthy adults, are uninsured by choice, preferring to use their monies for other purposes. Some are illegal immigrants, and some have recently lost their jobs and cannot afford to pay for benefits provided by the Consolidated Omnibus Budget Reconciliation Act (COBRA). Others are uninsured but eligible for such programs as the State Children's Health Insurance Program (SCHIP) or Medicaid. With such variation in the uninsured population, the answer will not be a one-size-fits-all solution.

Whether one believes in a government-sponsored and managed insurance system or not, it is unconscionable that the Untied States does not ensure catastrophic medical care for everyone and basic and preventive care for the less fortunate. I am well aware that it is far from a settled view in the United States, where there is great division concerning the government's role, especially in health care, and the public is ambivalent about taking care of the collective. That said, it is my belief that the question should not be *whether* everyone has a right to care but rather *how* to provide care to everyone in a cost-effective manner and in a fashion that expects a level of responsibility in return.

In an essay, Thomas Murray refers to Len Nichols, a senior member of the Health Policy Program at the New America Foundation in Washington, D.C. Nichols, he wrote,

> invoked the Old Testament. . . . Landowners are instructed in Leviticus: "When you reap the harvest of your land, you shall not reap to the very edges of your field, or gather the gleanings of your harvest; you shall leave them for the poor and the alien." The obligation is not limitless: the landowner does not have to prepare a meal, does not have to surrender the

entire crop, and should protect the land to ensure that it remains productive. But when food is more than sufficient to feed all, allowing some people to starve is indecent and represents a failure to live up to universal moral duties. To Nichols, the principle concerning the availability of food in Leviticus should be applied to health care today. . . . Stewardship requires us to be mindful of the basic needs of others and of the power and responsibility we have to use the resources in our control to meet those needs. Being a good steward for health care also requires that we use the community's resources wisely and well and that we protect and sustain them.[4]

It costs each of us today to have our fellow citizens uninsured. A sick person without insurance does not receive less expensive preventive care; instead, that person shows up at an emergency room seeking care. In the ER, care is more costly because the disease or illness has progressed further. Moreover, the ER is not designed for continuity of care. Primary care physicians are much better at addressing high blood pressure at its inception; diabetes at an early stage before vision, heart, or kidneys are damaged; and high cholesterol before it becomes a heart attack.

Many believe that Medicare is a good role model for health insurance. Not so. It has many drawbacks: It is expensive (see chapter 12), and despite taxing the income of all workers, it is heading toward bankruptcy. Medicare does not pay its fair share of expenses and attempts to control costs largely with price controls, which have consistently not worked. Finally, it has been equally consistently unwilling to innovate. In short, Medicare has not addressed the cost problem effectively; indeed, it has exacerbated it with its policies and approaches.

Insuring everyone means that it will cost us taxpayers more money. So it is absolutely imperative that we reduce the costs of medical care either before or as we attempt to expand insurance coverage for all in order that we do not further increase our medical care expenditures. This effort is just good stewardship of the limited resources available.

Lest this concept be construed as Pollyannaish dreaming, I acknowledge the process will not be simple and will take dollars up front to create a transition. Further, the effects of good preventive care will take years and quite probably generations to have maximal effect. But none of these observations are reason enough to postpone decisions and taking action.

Will health-care reform as legislated now accomplish this goal of providing medical care for all? It will prove to be a serious error if, in attempting to offer coverage to all, our political leaders let stand the old, tired, and ineffective current approach to insurance—be that government-sponsored or commercial programs. These systems have proven to offer less-than-adequate attention to prevention, screening, and care coordination while presiding over an inexorable rise in costs. It is imperative that we change the basic methodology. We need not only universal coverage and participation, but we must also give appropriate stewardship of the health-care resources we have.

We as individuals do not feel the real costs of medical care because, in most cases, we do not pay the first dollar; instead, our insurance does that, whether it be *moral hazard* commercial or government insurance. The president and Congress assured us that reform would mean that most Americans would notice little change. It was a logical statement for a politician to make, but if it is actually the case, then the reform is not what is actually needed.

The simple truth is that we cannot afford to give everyone everything. There is not enough money available to do so, no matter how much taxes are raised. We need to balance the generosity of the coverage with how much of the uninsured population will be given that coverage. Like it or not, choices will have to be made. It is probably far better to offer the greatest possible number of individuals a high-value policy—that is, a policy that protects against catastrophic problems and covers certain valuable preventive and basic services—rather than offer only some individuals complete and total prepaid medical care. At some point, the choices will have to be made, choices that politicians have wanted to avoid.[5]

Unfortunately, while there have been certain reforms of the insurance market, some nod to prevention programs, and a modicum of attention to expenditure management, the sad fact is that really critical elements needed for reform have not been addressed. Instead, new mandates, greater use of regulation, and frankly unaffordable new entitlements have been imposed.

THE PROPOSAL

First, we begin with the concept that everyone should have adequate medical care and that each of us needs to accept responsibility for our own health through diet, exercise, nutrition, seat belt use, dental hygiene, stress reduction, and tobacco avoidance.

We each also need to accept some level of first dollar payment for our medical care. Medical insurance years ago was for catastrophic needs such as hospitalization for a serious illness or surgery, but it has morphed into prepaid medical care for everything from routine visits, immunizations, and well-baby care to a host of well-meant but expensive mandates such as drugs and vaccines, mammograms, and colonoscopies. All of these measures are important to good health, but they should not necessarily be part of basic insurance.

The concept of insurance is to spread the risk of a less likely but high-cost event among many payers; thus, the insured pays a relatively low amount to provide for the catastrophic event that seldom occurs. Because medical insurance today is in actuality prepaid medical care that covers essentially everything and, unlike life insurance, does not allow for risk stratification, or adjustments to cover smoking and weight, medical insurance is expensive. Seventy percent of medical expenditures go for the care of those 10–15 percent of patients with serious, chronic diseases that last until death. Many cannot afford to pay out of pocket for the coordinated care these illnesses require, but insurance could cover PCP- or team-coordinated care.

We should move to a system where everyone can obtain insurance, as Congress mandated, but it should cover catastrophic needs, not routine needs. It will require a high deductible of, say, a thousand dollars or more. As with car collision insurance, the higher the deductible the lower the premium cost. And as with life insurance, medical insurance premiums should be based on age and lifestyle risk or behavior factors, such as weight and tobacco. But everyone, no matter their health status or preexisting condition, should have access. Further, everyone needs to be part of the pool so as to spread risk; no one should be allowed to opt out because they are young or their health is good. Currently, the individual mandate has been controversial, and will ultimately be addressed by the Supreme Court as to its constitutionality. Another approach, absent the mandate, would be to make insurance available to all despite preexisting conditions but with the proviso that the individual must show proof of having had coverage from another insurer within the prior six months.

This approach will mean a lower insurance bill, but it also will mean that each of us will pay for routine care up to a predetermined deductible. Since we will be paying for our basic care, we will be more likely to ask questions of our providers and determine whether a procedure is truly needed or a referral to a specialist will likely be useful. (It should be noted that a flat, thousand-dollar deductible incentivizes patients far differently than do multiple, small deductibles and co-pays. See my discussion of ulcers and of acid reflux in chapter 7 as an example. Our current deductible and co-pay arrangements create perverse incentives that actually encourage greater total expenditures rather than reducing them.)

Having medical savings accounts or health saving accounts to pay for routine care with pretax dollars makes this approach to out-of-pocket coverage of routine medical care more palatable and asks and encourages each of us to accept more responsibility for our care. If everyone has health insurance, our first dollar payments will be at the rate negotiated by the insurer. We will not be disadvantaged as if we did not have insurance and were self-pay patients who would get hit with a very high rate.

Every company should be required either to provide this type of insurance to its employees or to pay into a state or federal pool. For those individuals who cannot afford insurance, it should be subsidized either through tax credits or automatic enrollment in a government-sponsored plan akin to Medicare or the Federal Employee Health Benefit Plan (the former being both government paid and managed, the latter government paid but contracted out to commercial insurers). Those people who buy their insurance individually should have the same tax benefits as corporations do today. Since employees of businesses would be allowed to purchase their insurance directly with pretax dollars, then they should own the policy—not the employer—making it transportable from job to job, state to state, and even into retirement before Medicare kicks in.

For those who truly cannot afford basic care, insurance would cover the catastrophic problems, and government funds would support an HSA equivalent to pay for fundamentals: an annual exam; routine care; prevention strategies, such as recommended vaccines and critical screening tests; and a drug benefit generally focused on generics. This government-funded HSA would also cover programs to stop smoking, lose weight, learn about nutrition, and so on, with incentives to encourage participation and successful outcomes. The patient is still involved in the direct outlay of that first thousand-dollar deductible and will be more responsible for its use.

Commercial insurance should look at various models of coordinated care such as the CareFirst Blue Cross/Blue Shield contemplated program, which incents PCPs to give both preventive care and care coordination of chronic illness and which encourages health systems to have an orchestrator who will oversee care coordination for those with truly catastrophic illness. Medicare should be quick to embrace approaches similar to those of the Erickson Retirement Communities, which give unlimited primary care, added preventive care, chronic disease care coordination, and wellness and prevention management. These models provide better care at lower costs.[6] Insurers also need to change the current perverse incentives with co-pays that actually encourage using more expensive medications.

Understanding that most chronic illnesses area caused by adverse lifestyle behaviors, advocating wellness and prevention makes sense. The reform legislation did indeed change the Medicare reimbursement methodology such that every senior can have a paid-for annual wellness visit with his or her primary care physician, and most screening procedures that have been vetted are paid for as well. Commercial insurance will either need to pay for expanded wellness visits or need to be incented to do so beginning in 2014.

Like it or not, resources are not infinite. A new technology offering incremental benefit, but at high cost, will need to be considered in light of the total resources available. To call this analysis rationing is politically dangerous, but in fact, no matter the chosen terminology, relative resource allocations need to be made in medical care just as they are in all other aspects of life.

Businesses should follow the wellness models of companies like Safeway and General Mills that strive to improve health, reduce costs, and boost productivity. They should be allowed to benefit from changed laws that encourage the use of incentives to encourage their employees' effective participation.

The government, whether at the local, state, or federal level, might look to the Healthy Howard model, which helps those without insurance obtain good primary care, care coordination of chronic illness, and prescriptions with the help of a pharmacy benefits manager. In the process, Healthy Howard expects the individual to take responsibility by making modest payments and a change to a healthier lifestyle, with help from the program to overcome hurdles and barriers. As it expands coverage for all, the government also needs to create incentives that will encourage medical school graduates to enter primary care. One might take the form of loan forgiveness after a certain number of years of primary care practice.

Physicians have to be part of the solution. They must accept that it is their responsibility to provide high-quality preventive care for all and coordination for those with chronic illness. They must embrace the idea of working with other providers, such as nurse practitioners, and not try to marginalize them. They should look at what common procedures, tests, and referrals could be curtailed dramatically,[7] and they should consider how to prescribe in a more cost-effective manner. Doctors, especially primary care physicians, need to become orchestrators of care and not simply work as interveners as they do at present. To accomplish all of these goals, they will need to limit their practice to a truly manageable patient load (and insurance will need to adjust payment schedules so that incomes stay about the same). Physicians and hospitals will need to find ways to work together effectively for the patient's benefit, and for each episode of care they will agree to accept a global fee to be divided among all involved in an equitable fashion. All parties need to be held accountable for observing evidence-based, proven practices whether that be routine hand washing or avoiding expensive procedures that have been demonstrated as useless. Physicians need to be real leaders in reducing adverse events and improving the quality of care. In effect, this represents a shift from a service orientation to an outcome orientation, as well as a shift from a provider-centric to a patient-centric model of care.

We individuals need to be part of the solution as well. Unlike when we make other purchases, we often act irrationally in relation to health-care decisions because we are uninformed or we make decisions based on emotional responses rather than after intellectual consideration. We tend to choose those things that we think will be helpful or important. Some egregious examples occur as a patient nears the end of life and overuses medical care. Less egregious, but unfortunate, is using funds to meet an insurance deductible to purchase a suggested test or procedure that is likely not needed and then not having the necessary funds later to obtain solid primary care.

In another aspect of making medical care more cost effective, medical liability must have caps for pain and suffering, and settlement should be by a nonjudicial tribunal or a special court. The expectation will be for prompt explanation, apology, and payment for harm followed by root cause analysis and corrective action to prevent similar errors in the future. Physicians will be held accountable for any gross lapses in safety and face exclusion from the operating room or hospital admission privileges for a period that is sufficient to create a financial incentive for proper practice.

The federal government will establish (and the reform legislation has so mandated) a quasi-independent organization or institute to evaluate technologies, drugs, devices, equipment, and care protocols. Its board should be comprised of highly regarded physicians of impeccable reputation who are appointed for lengthy, staggered terms. This board could make use of nonprofit organizations and professional societies that are already engaged in legitimate evidence-based reviews for some of its evaluations. The findings should be published widely and posted on the Internet for the patients' and the providers' review alike. Insurers should not use the results to deny payment if a physician presents credible reasons why an individual patient might benefit from a prescribed treatment although it was found ineffectual when evaluated for a large group. Individual patients' circumstances may occasionally, but not often, trump group averages.

This combination of rights and responsibilities can ensure everyone access to care and incentives to better health. Yet, it will reduce expenditures and eliminate many of the frustrations with the current system. Many of the proposed steps are small steps, but when added together, they can have a large impact. It is a plan that satisfies both legitimate arguments—that medical care is a right and that we all must accept a meaningful level of responsibility for our health and its costs. And it will mean a real and lasting stewardship of our limited yet critical resources.

It is important at this junction to state once again that this transition will not be easy or rapid. There are myriad obstacles and many interested parties that will look to preserve what they believe is important to them. It will mean a new medical care culture, and cultural change is never easy. But with enlightened leadership, the transition can be made.

What will be the results?

Everyone is insured. The risks will be spread over the entire population, those who choose to engage in high-risk behavior such as smoking will pay a higher rate, no one will be denied coverage, and those truly unable to pay will be covered by the government, either through tax credits or a direct subsidy. It will meet both the Democrats' desire to ensure universal coverage and the Republicans' desire to require greater personal responsibility and use market forces to reduce costs. At the same time, the approaches suggested to improve quality and safety will have a major impact on reducing the costs of care. This approach will bring relief to businesses, the federal and state governments, and the average citizen who pays for both the high cost of care and the high taxes needed to deliver it to the less fortunate. Since we will pay for routine and predictable care needs out of pocket with tax-advantaged HSAs, we will begin to monitor the costs and necessity of the tests, procedures, and referrals that our providers suggest. Those who must depend on the government to fund their HSAs will become informed purchasers also since the HSAs will only cover so much. Most important, it will mean that patients with complicated illnesses will get the care and coordination of care that they need and deserve from physicians who will have limited the size of their practice to accommodate the time required for good preventive care and chronic illness care coordination. Finally, a good federal program that focuses the country on meaningful prevention strategies, including changing our own lifestyles, will reap huge payoffs into the future as will augmentation of public health services in general.

Members of both parties could take great pride in reaching such a compromise for added reform elements because it would serve everyone with better care, improve the overall health of the nation, and reduce skyrocketing expenditures. Misconceptions can be converted to expectations for a better future. What an incredible outcome for all.

---
17 —

What You Can Do to Get Quality Care and Keep Your Costs Down

Misconception: *I cannot do very much to prevent disease as I get older; it all depends on my doctor or what is in my genes.*

Is this you? You have a good job. You have done well and see opportunities for a promotion in the future. But it is hard work, requires many extra hours, and causes stress. You have a nice family that you love dearly, but you have relatively little time with them. You are overweight—not obese—and you know it would be good to lose that ten to twenty pounds. Knowing you do not get enough exercise, you actually bought a membership to a health club about six months ago, but you cannot remember the last time you were there.

This morning you need to get to work early, so you skip breakfast and stop at a coffee shop for a mocha latte and a blueberry scone to eat in the car while driving to work. Lunch will be something picked up from a fast-food outlet and possibly even eaten at your desk. There will not be time to cook dinner tonight so you will, one more time, order carryout. You know it would be nice to have the whole family sit down together for dinner, but that is just not practical. Besides, right after supper is over, you need to go pick up your older child from soccer practice. You are thinking that there simply is not enough time to spend with your family but perhaps this weekend . . . but not until you make some progress made on that big presentation that you will be making on Monday morning.

Does the person in the story above sound in any way like you? The simple fact is that many of us resemble that person, and our lifestyles portend chronic disease later in life. But the good news is now you know it, and you can do something about it.

As I wrote in *The Future of Medicine*, "We can put all the advances from science and technology to our benefit—to help prevent illness and to treat it when it occurs. But it is equally important that we do take good care of the body we have been entrusted with. That is our own personal obligation. No doctor or nurse or procedure or pill can do that for us."

You can make a difference. Remember, it is much easier to live a reasonably healthy lifestyle than it is to fix a damaged body. It is never too late to start. Your body will love you for it. It is not hard, but it does take some time each and every day. Enjoy your health in the knowledge that if you keep your body and mind at peak performance, then with the fruits of the new medical megatrends and the help of your health-care providers, you will be able to make remarkable inroads when you are injured or develop a serious disease.

Here I will summarize the book's salient conclusions and offer a plan for maintaining your own health and controlling your own costs.

From my research that I did in preparation for this book, we can now also look at how medical care should be *delivered* in the coming years. We have learned that instead of a focus on health care and prevention, we have a medical care system that concentrates on diseases, most research addresses illness, and our payment systems are clearly directed toward illness. With our aging population, there will be more illnesses to treat that will be lifelong, complex, chronic conditions rather than the more acute and limited illnesses of the past. Our medical care will need to change from its current uncoordinated, medical discipline–based approach to a patient-centric, disease-based approach with well-coordinated team-based care that incorporates disease management, care management, and wellness management. Primary care physicians will need to become orchestrators of care rather than be the interventionalists that they are at present, and with only 30 percent of all practicing physicians today, we must encourage more physicians to become PCPs. They are the key not only to care coordination but also to ensuring good preventive care as well. Nurse practitioners, physician assistants, pharmacists, nurses, social workers, optometrists, and others will need to be afforded greater opportunities to participate in the medical care system. We will need to take ownership of our medical records and insist that we be given copies of reports after every encounter, especially until an electronic medical record is universally available. Further, if we don't want costs to continue to increase rapidly, we will need insurance payments to change and create incentives for ensuring good care coordination and preventive interventions and for all of us to lead healthier lifestyles.

As the interaction of medicine with computer science and engineering rapidly advances, medical technologies of life-saving, life-altering, and life-improving value will emerge at an increasingly fast rate. Other drivers of the changes in medical care will be the rise of consumerism. Patients simply no longer will be willing to be "patient." Patients directly, and through hospital trustees and various agencies, will insist on quality and safety in every aspect of medical care and practice. But professional shortages of physicians, especially generalists, along with nurses, pharmacists, and others, will mean that access to care, especially in rural and urban poor areas, will suffer even further. Others will either refuse to participate in Medicare or Medicaid or opt for retainer-based practices with fewer patients so that they can assure themselves and their patients of having adequate time and attention.

Patients will be expected to take on greater responsibility for maintaining their health and paying for their care. All of these drivers of change will mean more hospitals; more beds, especially in intensive care units; and more highly sophisticated operating rooms. Technology will be of greater importance to medical care, with more medical devices, such as pacemakers, having a major impact. Yet, concurrently medicine must get back to its roots and tradition with closer personal interaction between patients and provider. New biomedical science—such as genomics, stem cells, and nanotechnology—will greatly influence patient care. And finally, safety and quality will not be mere slogans but will become the essence of medical care.

But important changes in the *delivery* of health care must occur if we are to benefit from the profound advances in biomedical and engineering sciences. Our system of health care must evolve and offer more preventive care, wellness care, and health promotion. We as patients will need incentives to adjust our behaviors and maintain our health. Providers also will need incentives to offer team-based care, care coordination, and disease management rather than the current approach of individual providers working on a pay-for-visit or pay-for-encounter basis. Improved care coordination is absolutely essential if those with complex, chronic diseases are to obtain the top-notch quality of care that our knowledge and technology can provide in an effective, efficient, and satisfying manner. We need rapid, easy access to primary care providers, which will mean offering incentives for more physicians to enter primary care. Primary care providers will need a payment system that encourages their spending adequate time with their patients.

Certainly, we also need a simplified financing system with less paperwork, less bureaucracy, and less money wasted on activities that do not deliver care. I believe we should return to an insurance system that covers major or catastrophic needs while we individuals pay out of pocket (with monies from a tax-advantaged HSAs) for routine and preventive care. As we accept more personal responsibility for our health and for our health care, our insurance should be tiered so that we pay more if we persist in our health-adverse habits, like smoking and obesity, but no one should be denied coverage because of a preexisting condition. Everyone should be required to purchase the basic coverage for expensive or catastrophic care.

We must bring health-care costs down. Indeed, I believe that this goal should have been the first priority of health-care reform. Costs are rising for many reasons including a shift from caring for acute illnesses to ones that are lifelong, chronic, and complex to treat; insufficient attention to patient safety; the overuse of procedures, new technologies, and drugs, the poor coordination of care of chronic illness; our poor personal behaviors; and the aging of the population, which suffers more diseases.

Bringing down the costs of care will not be easy, but understanding the causes gives us a place to start. We need to start with care coordination, disease prevention, and wellness promotion. We need a coordinated, integrated, and comprehensive approach that will address, one by one, all of the barriers to implementation. Of particular importance is care coordination by primary care physicians for those with chronic illness and organized teams of providers for those with catastrophic illnesses. This arrangement is critical and essential if we want to ensure quality and safety and reduce costs. Patients, businesses, and governments as payers can benefit from these improvements since enhanced quality will bring down the expenditures. The key step is to create monetary incentives for physicians to spend the time necessary for thorough care coordination and connect those incentives to actual requirements that the patient's care is in fact coordinated. Again, the approach melds rights with responsibilities. Finally, we need to change insurance so that the individual can purchase it with tax-advantaged dollars, purchase a high-deductible policy with fewer mandates, and have an HSA to pay for basic, predictable care needs.

After taking the steps suggested in this book, it will be possible to rewrite the "many misconceptions" about health care as health care's "many results." We *can* have true health care and not simply medical care. We also can offer access to all. Adding new people to the roles of the insured will be expensive, but concurrently, to offset those costs, we can reduce both the cost of care substantially and the burden on individuals, businesses, and governments. The cost of care can come down and the quality and the safety of care go up while the time providers spend directly with their patients can be increased. Thus, America can have the best system of health-care delivery to go with its status as having the best medical research and development. In short, we can have a system of care delivery worthy of world emulation.

TO YOUR GOOD HEALTH

Meanwhile, here is what you can do now to keep your own health-care costs as low as possible while still enjoying good health and getting excellent care. Start by finding a good primary care physician, probably an internist or a family medicine physician, for yourself and a pediatrician for your children. Interview doctors until you find someone who is compatible with your needs and your personality. You might want to look for one who has a retainer-based practice or one who charges by the hour, has a limited number of patients, and will offer you as much time per visit as you decide you need and are willing to pay for. Then be sure to get an annual evaluation, and before going to a specialist for a problem, check with your PCP first. In all likelihood, the PCP can solve your problem. If not, asking the PCP for his or her recommendation for a specialist is probably the way to go. Physicians like to refer to other doctors who they have learned over the years are responsive to their patients, get back to them with recommendations, and, of course, are well trained and up to date. Ask your PCP to personally contact the specialist and explain the reasons for the referral; and ask the specialist to return the favor after examining you. This will markedly improve information transfer and hence your care.

If any doctor suggests a test, X-ray, or procedure, be sure to ask exactly why it is proposed and what the doctor hopes to learn from the test. Will the information really be useful? Or is it being ordered to be "complete"? If you are prescribed a drug, ask if a cheaper, generic formulation is available.

Whenever you visit a doctor, come prepared. It is always a good idea to write down a list of the most important issues you want to discuss. Begin with the most pressing one first, and don't wait to raise it until the doctor starts to leave the examining room. Do your own homework on the Internet by gathering information from reputable websites such as those listed in the Resources Section. Come to your doctor's office with questions based on your studies.

Talk to your physician about what preventive measures you should be taking—immunizations, vitamins, and more—and then follow that advice. Look at your own behaviors. Do you smoke? Are you overweight? Do you sometimes drive after drinking? Do you talk or text on a cell phone while driving? Do you take good care of your teeth? Get help where you need it, say for quitting smoking. It will be money well spent. And, since most insurance does not pay for most preventive medicine, be prepared to pay for it yourself. It will pay you back manyfold. Check whether your employer offers wellness programs; if it does not, suggest that it consider them. If it does, use them as appropriate to your situation.

Be sure to see other health-care providers as well. You should see your dentist regularly and get a dental cleaning, or prophylaxis, twice a year, because dental caries and periodontal disease are major causes not only of local disease but also systemic disease. Be sure your water supply is fluoridated because this mineral has been well documented to markedly reduce cavities. If your PCP does not do vision or hearing exams, be sure to see an optometrist or ophthalmologist every two years. If you are nearing retirement age, a hearing test is a good idea.

Finally, ask for—insist if necessary—a copy of your records after a visit, for a CD of your X-ray, CT scan, or MRI; and a copy of your hospital record when discharged. (You will probably have to pay a small fee for the hospital record.) These records will be invaluable if you are required to see a specialist in a distant city since the specialist will expect you to bring all of the relevant information. Keep a list of your medications and preferably carry a duplicate in your wallet or purse along with your physician's phone number. It will prove handy if you must visit an ER, have an accident, or become ill while traveling.

Should you develop a chronic disease, talk to your primary care physician and request good care coordination. Be prepared and offer to pay for it. Also, be sure that your PCP realizes that you know what you are talking about, that you know what you want, and that you are absolutely serious about it. If you have a challenging problem that requires your referral to a major medical center, go to one that employs the team-based, multidisciplinary approach to coordinated care. Ask many questions. Do not accept anything less. Advocating for yourself is critical to ensure you get the best medical care.

It is your body, so protect it by obtaining the best care that is available. If you do so, your care will be improved, and your medical care costs will be much lower. More important, you will be much healthier, and you will enjoy life more.

America is a remarkable country whose citizens have enormous ingenuity and a generous spirit. Putting these two characteristics together should—or at least could—allow us to bring down the costs of care and at the same time ensure everyone has excellent and safe care, care that is truly health care and not merely medical care. This goal is doable and doable now. If we are successful, our world-class care will set the standard for other countries to emulate.

ACKNOWLEDGMENTS

Many people helped bring this book to fruition. They gave generously of their time and their knowledge.

A section of this book on the Hospital of the Future was developed in part thorough a consulting contract with the Telemedicine and Advanced Technology Research Center (TATRC) of the U.S. Army at Fort Detrick in Frederick, Maryland, where I was afforded access to numerous physicians, nurses, and others engaged in advancing medical technologies both at TATRC and through their partners and collaborators across the country. Special thanks go to Amy Nyswaner, RN; Col. Karl Friedl; Col. Ron Poropatich; Col. Hon Pak; and Dr. Charles Peterson. This work was bolstered by an opportunity to interact with the American Hospital Association's Long-Range Planning Committee as it tried to determine what the future might hold for its member hospitals and by presentations and participation in a meeting at the Institute of Medicine regarding future hospital design criteria.

I interviewed more than 150 people across the country who were exceptionally generous with their time and willingly shared their expertise. I cannot name them all here, but please know that you are appreciated.

Margaret Frazier took my dictations and converted them to the written word, always with a smile. She made numerous corrections, edited the references, and in general kept me on track. Nancy Johnson markedly improved my grammar and sentence structure.

Richard Knapp, retired executive vice president and chief advocacy officer of the Association of American Medical Colleges, and Frank Samuels reviewed the entire manuscript. James Bentley, retired senior vice president of the American Hospital Association; Don McDaniel Jr., CEO of Sage Growth Partners; James Kagen, consulting director with the Chartis Group; Vivian Reifberg, partner in McKinsey & Company; Mathew Narrett, MD, executive vice president and chief medical officer of Erickson Health; Jerome Carr, JD, chief of compliance and legal affairs for University Physicians, Inc.; Donald N. Joyce, administrator, specialty practices, Providence Hospital; Keith Persinger and Harold Standiford, MD, chief financial officer and hospital epidemiologist, respectively, of the University of Maryland Medical Center—all have reviewed one or more chapters of the manuscript. Chet Burrell, CEO of CareFirst Blue Cross/Blue Shield; Marshall Steele, MD; and Ken Ulman, Howard County (Maryland) Executive, reviewed sections of chapters. I owe each of them a special thank-you. Despite all of this assistance, any remaining errors are mine alone.

My literary agent, Cynthia Zigmund, was a source of valuable ideas, encouragement, and commitment. The staff at Potomac has been equally committed to making this book as excellent as possible, including publisher Sam Dorrance, acquisition editor Hilary Claggett, production editor Julie Gutin, and copyeditor Vicki Chamlee.

Special thanks go to my wife of forty-eight years, Carol Schimpff, who not only tolerated my idiosyncrasies, but also helped me immeasurably to think through issues, to connect with the most useful sources of information, and to keep me focused on the final product. As a retired architect, MBA, and watercolorist, she showed a creativity combined with business sense that were invaluable. She had patience when I did not and offered me warm support at all times.

To all of you, I acknowledge your assistance and offer my sincere thanks.

NOTES

Chapter 1. The Difference between Health Care and Medical Care

1. "Health Care Spending in the United States and Selected OECD Countries, April 2011," Kaiser Family Foundation, http://www.kff.org/insurance/snapshot/OECD042111.cfm (accessed September 12, 2011).

Chapter 2. What Really Needs to Change

1. Steven Schroeder, MD, "We Can Do Better—Improving the Health of the American People," *New England Journal of Medicine* 357 (2007): 1221–28.

2. J. C. Murray and J. Frank, "Ranking 37th—Measuring the Performance of the U.S. Healthcare System," *New England Journal of Medicine* 362 (2010): 98–99.

3. J. M. Gaziano, "Fifth Phase of the Epidemiologic Transition: The Age of Obesity and Inactivity," *Journal of the American Medical Association* 303 (2010): 275–76.

4. "The Global Economic Burden of Noncommunicable Diseases," World Economic Forum, Harvard School of Public Health, September 2011, http://www3.weforum.org/docs/WEF_Harvard_HE_GlobalEconomicBurdenNonCommunicableDiseases_2011.pdf (accessed September 19, 2011).

5. Ross DeVol and Armen Bedroussian, "An Unhealthy America: The Economic Impact of Chronic Disease," the Milken Institute, 2007, http://www.milkeninstitute.org/pdf/chronic_disease_report.pdf (accessed September 19, 2011).

6. Ibid.

7. Peter Orszag and Philip Ellis, Addressing Rising Health Care Costs—a View from the Congressional Budget Office," *New England Journal of Medicine* 357 (2007): 1885–87.

8. Modified from Allan Sloan, "Ahoy, Blackstone, and Ready the Harpoons," *Washington Post*, April 3, 2007.

Chapter 3. What Change Looks Like: A Vision for the Future

1. The argument against this approach is that I won't have any incentive to obtain the necessary preventive care if I have to pay for it out of pocket. There are many approaches to consider such as reduced insurance costs if I don't smoke, do exercise, and do have an appropriate weight and if I show evidence of obtaining such preventive or screening tests as blood pressure and cholesterol measurements. Certainly we also need to accept that we each have to take responsibility for our own health, and that concern might include a financial cost, personal time, and attention.

2. "Health Care Spending in the United States and Selected OECD Countries, April 2011," Kaiser Family Foundation.

3. Kristine Gebbie, Linda Rosenstock, and Lyla M. Hernandez, *eds.*, *Who Will Keep the Public Healthy? Educating Public Health Professionals for the 21st Century* (Washington, DC: Institute of Medicine, November 4, 2002).

Chapter 4. Scientific Advances That Will Affect Health Care—with or without Reform

1. When I attended Yale Medical School forty-plus years ago, there were few women in the class. The year before I graduated in 1967 was the first year that a woman had been accepted as a surgical resident at Yale New Haven Hospital. Today, about half of medical school graduates are women, and they enter any specialty. Indeed, a woman is now chief of surgery at Johns Hopkins.

2. These megatrends in science were discussed in detail in my earlier book, *The Future of Medicine: Megatrends in Health Care That Will Improve Your Quality of Life* (Nashville, TN: Thomas Nelson, 2007).

Chapter 5. Surprising Drivers of Change in Health-Care Delivery

1. As a necessity, much of medicine needs to be organized and operated like a business. But unlike a business where profit is the key end point, the purpose of the medical profession is to improve health and treat disease. Physicians constantly need to put the needs of their patients in front of their own financial gain (or that of hospitals, surgicenters, etc.). Health care is a major industry with pharmaceutical and device companies focused on making profits for their shareholders, for-profit insurers doing the same, and not-for-profit hospitals, of necessity, focused on a strong net income each year to reinvest in the facility and in technologies. In this environment, many physicians begin to think and then act as though business considerations come first. This behavior pattern has and is continuing to change the face of medical professionalism. For a deeper analysis, refer to an article by Dr Arnold Relman, "Medical Professionalism in a Commercialized Health Care Market," *Journal of the American Medical Association* 298 (2007): 2668–69.

2. A. Jha et al., "Patients' Perception of Hospital Care in the United States," *New England Journal of Medicine* 359 (2008): 1921–31.

3. R. Voelker, "US Health Care System Earns Poor Marks," *Journal of the American Medical Association* 300, no. 24 (2008): 2843–44, which in turn cited C. Schoen, et al., "In Chronic Condition: Experience of Patients with Complex Health Care Needs in Eight Countries," *Health Affairs*, November 13, 2008.

4. Personal communication, B. H. Johnson, Institute for Family-Centered Care, February 2010.

5. Association of American Medical Colleges, https://www.aamc.org (accessed September 12, 2011).

6. P. I. Buerhaus, "Current and Future State of the US Nursing Workforce," *Journal of the American Medical Association* 300 (2008): 2422–24.

Chapter 6. The Tsunami Is Coming

1. S. P. Phillips and E. B. Austin, "The Feminization of Medicine and Population Health," *Journal of the American Medical Association* 301 (2009): 863–64.

2. For a fuller discussion, see chapter 9 on complementary medicine in my book *The Future of Medicine*.

3. For a more detailed exposition of these concepts, review R. M. S. Bohmer's "Fixing Health Care on the Front Lines" (62–69), and T. H. Lee's "Turning Doctors into Leaders" (50–59), both in *Harvard Business Review*, April 2010.

4. For an in-depth discussion of alignment in academic medical centers, see Morton Rapoport and Stephen Schimpff, *Alignment: The Key to the Success of the University of Maryland Medical System* (Baltimore: University of Maryland Medical System, 2009).

5. As I discuss in chapter 5, physicians now prefer being employed, often by a hospital, rather than be in private practice. My statement here that most practicing physicians are not in the hospital employ is undergoing a major upheaval.

Chapter 7. Health-Care Financing: Basic Concepts

1. V. D. Hayes, "A Premium Sucker Punch," *Washington Post*, January 25, 2009; and based on data from the Kaiser Family Foundation and the Health Research and Education Trust. Employer Health benefits, 2010, Exhibit 1, page 1, http://ehbs.kff.org/pdf/2010/8086.pdf (accessed September 13, 2011).

2. Figures derived from the Kaiser Family Foundation, "Health Care Costs: A Primer," http://ehbs.kff.org/pdf/2010/8086.pdf (accessed September 13, 2011).

3. M. Hartman et al., "National Health Spending in 2007, Slower Drug Spending Contributes to Lowest Rate of Overall Growth Since 1998," *Health Affairs* 28 (2009): 246–61.

4. Figures derived from the Kaiser Family Foundation, "Health Care Costs: A Primer."

5. I would be inclined to label obesity as a behavior or at least as a result of behaviors (overeating and too little exercise), and not as a disease, per se. But it is the proximate cause of many diseases such as heart disease and type 2 diabetes, and it makes many others worse. For example, a person with osteoarthritis who becomes obese puts even further stress on damaged knees.

6. Steven A. Burd, "How Safeway Is Cutting Health-Care Costs," Op-Ed, *Wall Street Journal*, June 12, 2009.

7. McKinsey Global Institute, "Accounting for the Cost of US Health Care: A New Look at Why Americans Spend More," *McKinsey and Company*, December 2008.

8. "Dartmouth Atlas of Health Care," http://www.dartmouthatlas.org/. The data used in the text come from their report entitled "Health Care Spending, Quality and Outcomes," found at http://www.dartmouthatlas.org/downloads/reports/Spending_Brief_022709.pdf. In addition, the site has many very useful reports, the most recent being at http://www.dartmouthatlas.org/downloads/reports/EOL_Trend_Report_0411.pdf (accessed September 13, 2011).

Chapter 8. The Real Reason Why Our Health-Care Costs Keep Going Up

1. F. J. Crosson, "21st Century Health Care: The Case for Integrated Delivery Systems," *New England Journal of Medicine* 361 (2009): 1324–25.

2. D. Peikes et al., "Effects of Care Coordination on Hospitalization, Quality of Care and Health Care Expenditures among Medicare Beneficiaries: 15 Randomized Trials," *Journal of the American Medical Association* 301 (2009): 603–18.

3. J. Z. Ayanian, "The Elusive Quest for Quality and Cost Savings in the Medicare Program," *Journal of the American Medical Association* 301 (2009): 668–70.

4. John Erickson, personal communication, February and June 2009.

5. P. R. Nader et al., "Moderate-to-Vigorous Physical Activity from Ages 9 to 15 Years," *Journal of the American Medical Association* 300 (2008): 295–305.

6. A. H. Mokdad et al., "Actual Causes of Death in the United States, 2000," *Journal of the American Medical Association*, 291, no. 10 (2004): 1238–45.

7. Steven Burd, "How Safeway Is Cutting Health-Care Costs." with updated information via email from Brian Dowling at Safeway on February 23, 2011.

8. E. C. Schimpff, http://radishboy.blogspot.com (accessed June 26, 2011).

9. S. H. Woolf, "A Closer Look at the Economic Argument for Disease Prevention," *Journal of the American Medical Association* 301 (2009): 536–38.

10. For a good discussion, see Michael Pollan, *In Defense of Food: An Eater's Manifesto* (New York: Penguin Press, 2008).

11. See my description of a measles outbreak among unvaccinated children in home schools in *The Future of Medicine*, 56–57.

Chapter 9. The High Cost of Drugs and Technologies

1. Institute of Medicine, Committee on Comparative Effectiveness Research Priori-

tization, *Initial National Priorities for Comparative Effectiveness Research* (Washington, DC: National Academy of Sciences, 2009).

Chapter 13. The Looming Crisis in Primary Care

1. K Grumbach, "Redesign of the Health Care Delivery System: A Bauhaus 'Form Follows Function' Approach," *Journal of the American Medical Association* 302, no. 21 (2009): 2363–64.

2. D. R. Rittenhouse, S. M. Shortell, and E. S. Fisher, "Primary Care and Accountable Care—Two Essential Elements of Delivery System Reform," *New England Journal of Medicine* 361 (2009): 2301–3.

3. E. Hargrave et al., *Retainer Based Physicians: Characteristics, Impact and Policy Considerations,* http://medpac.gov/documents/Oct10_RetainerBasedPhysicians _CONTRACTOR_CB.pdf (accessed September 18, 2011).

4. Team-based care began at the cancer center in the early 1980s when Dr. Joseph Aisner, then the clinical director, suggested to me that we begin a weekly session for women with known or suspected breast cancer in which the surgeon, medical oncologist, and radiation oncologist all would see each new patient together with the breast cancer nurse practitioner. The radiologist and the pathologist would be available for immediate consultation. We could only bill for one of the three physicians, so I agreed to cover the other physicians with institutional funds in a sort of "loss leader" arrangement. It was an immediate success; patients were very pleased and so were the providers. Later this approach became the standard way the University of Maryland Greenebaum Cancer Center functioned for all patients, and it led to the construction of an outpatient facility designed especially for team-based care, funded specifically for this purpose through a gift of Leonard and Rosalyn Stoler, who believed in this style of care.

5. When the surgical team has a brief discussion in the OR, immediately before starting the operation, they are doing the same thing—that is, bringing all the issues to the forefront among the surgeon, nurse, and anesthesiologist when it most matters. The care is better, errors are much less likely to occur, and the team members feel better for the effort. The Veterans Health Administration (as cited in an article by J. Neiley et al., "Association Between Implementation of a Medical Team Training Program and Surgical Mortality," *Journal of the American Medical Association,* 304, no. 15 [2010]: 1693–1700) has mandated this type of briefing in their 130 hospitals that perform surgery. They have seen a reduction in operative mortality as a result.

Chapter 14. Some Final Thoughts on Cost Management

1. Melinda Beeuwkes et al., "Healthcare Spending and Preventive Care in High-Deductible and Consumer-Driven Health Plans," *American Journal of Managed*

Care 17 (2011): 222–30. A summary can be found at http://www.eurekalert.org/pub_releases/2011-03/rc-lso032211.php (accessed September 21, 2011).

2.   Aetna website, http://www.aetna.com/about-aetna-insurance/public-policy-per spectives/consumer-directed-health-care.html (accessed September 21, 2011).

Chapter 15. What Reform Looks Like: Differing Views

1.   T. A. Murray, "American Values and Health Care Reform," *New England Journal of Medicine* 362 (2010): 285–87.

2.   M. G. Bloche, "Health Care for All," *New England Journal of Medicine* 357 (2007): 1173–75.

3.   Oberlander used data from the Kaiser Family foundation health tracking poll of August 2007, available at http://www.kff.org/kaiserpolls/upload/7691.pdf (accessed September 17, 2011).

4.   J. Oberlander, "Presidential Politics and the Resurgence of Health Care Reform," *New England Journal of Medicine* 357 (2007): 2101–4.

5.   The October 2008 Kaiser Family Foundation health tracking poll can be found at http://www.kff.org/kaiserpolls/upload/7832.pdf (accessed September 17, 2011).

6.   The December 2009 Kaiser Family Foundation health tracking poll can be found at http://www.kff.org/kaiserpolls/upload/8037.pdf (accessed September 17, 2011).

7.   The March 2010 Kaiser Family Foundation health tracking poll can be found at http://www.kff.org/kaiserpolls/8058.cfm (accessed September 17, 2011).

8.   Tom Daschle with S. S. Greenberger and J. M. Lambrew, *Critical: What We Can Do about the Health-Care Crisis* (New York: St. Martin's Griffin/Thomas Dunne Books, 2009).

9.   D. .F Kallmes et al., "A Randomized Trial of Vertebroplasty for Osteoporotic Spinal Fractures," *New England Journal of Medicine,* 361 (2009): 569–79.

10. Atul Gawande, "Getting There from Here: How Should Obama Reform Health Care?" *New Yorker,* January 26, 2009, 26–33.

11. Health tracking poll from Kaiser Family foundation for August 2011 available at http://www.kff.org/kaiserpolls/upload/8217-F.pdf (accessed September 17, 2011).

12. There are many sources that summarize the Patient Protection and Affordable Care Act, among them are the official government website http://www.health-care.gov/law/introduction/index.html, a summary prepared by Senate Democrats at http://dpc.senate.gov/healthreformbill/healthbill04.pdf, and a well-done overview with interactive sections by the Kaiser Family Foundation at http://health reform.kff.org/. See also the excellent book prepared by the staff of the *Washington Post* noted in the Resources section of this book.

Chapter 16. Recommendations for Reform:
Aligning Rights with Responsibilities

1.   David Hilzenrath, "Misleading Claims about Safeway Wellness Incentives Shape Health-Care Bill," *Washington Post,* January 17, 2010.

2. Kevin G. Volpp et al., "Redesigning Employee Health Incentives—Lessons from Behavioral Economics," *New England Journal of Medicine* 365 (2011): 388–90.

3. Richard H. Thaler and Cass R. Sunstein, *Nudge: Improving Decisions about Health, Wealth, and Happiness* (New Haven, CT: Yale University Press, 2008).

4. Murray, "American Values and Health Care Reform."

5. K. Baicker and A. Chandra, "Uncomfortable Arithmetic—Whom to Cover versus What to Cover," *New England Journal of Medicine* 362 (2010): 95–97. The premise is based on an article by Dr. Howard Brody (see note 5 of this chapter).

6. Medicare would benefit from a board of experts, mostly physicians with wide experience, that could make recommendations for payment adjustments and alterations, such as paying for care coordination, enhanced bundling of service payments, and so forth. Such a group was established as part of the Affordable Care Act, but it is not clear that the board will have the flexibility to make the types of recommendations actually needed to lower costs while maintaining quality, coverage and benefits. This Board is different from the Federal Coordinating Council for Comparative Effectiveness Research that was mandated by the American Reinvestment and Recovery act (the "stimulus" bill). This Council is made up of 15 members, all from various federal agencies, charged to coordinate research and guide the allocated $1.1 billion investments in this endeavor. By its charter, the Council will "provide information on the relative strengths and weakness of various medical interventions" but will "not recommend clinical guidelines for payment, coverage or treatment." More information can be found at http://www.hhs.gov/recovery/programs/os/cerbios.html.

7. See Dr. Howard Brody, "Medicine's Ethical Responsibility for Health Care Reform—the Top Five List," *New England Journal of Medicine* 362 (2010): 283–85, where he suggests every medical specialty produce a list of five procedures that are common and costly, yet of limited usefulness. Examples might include routine MRIs for low back pain, antibiotic prescriptions for pharyngitis likely to be caused by a virus, and thyroid tests for asymptomatic patients. This list could become long, and it should. Physicians need to take responsibility and demonstrate that they, too, are serious about cost management. It is good stewardship of scarce and costly resources. This piece was followed by Dr. Thomas Smith and Dr. Bruce Hillner's "Bending the Cost Curve in Cancer Care," *New England Journal of Medicine* 362 (May 26, 2011): 21. These two medical oncologists wrote cogently about what could be done in medical oncology that would markedly reduce costs yet at the same time substantially improve quality. But their proposals will affect their fellow oncologists' pocketbook, so acceptance, unfortunately, is unlikely.

RESOURCES

Listed here are books, journals, organizations, and websites that give further information related to the issues, concepts, and topics in this book.

Books

Shannon Brownlee. *Overtreated: Why Too Much Medicine Is Making Us Sicker and Poorer.* New York: Bloomsbury USA, 2007.

> Ms Brownlee, a health and medical writer and acting director of the New America Foundation Health Policy Program, gives data suggesting that as much as one-third of health-care expenditures are for unnecessary specialist visits, procedures, tests, and prescriptions. Her finding is consistent with the observations I make in part 3 of this volume. She lays the blame on a "national delusion" that more care is better care.

Clayton Christensen, Jerome H. Grossman, and John Hwang. *The Innovator's Prescription: A Disruptive Solution for Health Care.* New York: McGraw-Hill, 2008.

> Christensen, a professor at the Harvard Business School, has written extensively about innovation and entrepreneurship. The late Dr. Grossman was CEO of the New England Medical Center for sixteen years in Boston. Dr. Hwang is an internist and executive director of health care at Innosight Institute, a nonprofit social innovation think tank based in Mountain View, California. In this book the trio make recommendations on "precision medicine" to reduce costs and improve quality, propose a variety of disruptive business models to change the way doctors and hospitals do their work, and show how employers can change their roles in health care to compete more effectively.

Tom Daschle. *Critical: What We Can Do about the Health-Care Crisis.* With Scott S. Greenberger and Jeanne M. Lambrew. New York: St. Martin's Griffin/Thomas Dunne Books, 2008.

> Former senator Daschle and his colleagues describe their vision for health-care reform, including the creation of a national board, modeled on the Federal Reserve concept, to review evidence-based information. In many ways, the health-reform legislation was modeled on Daschle's concepts.

Atul Gawande. *The Checklist Manifesto: How to Get Things Right.* New York: Henry Holt/Metropolitan Books, 2009.

> Dr. Gawande, an oncologic surgeon at Harvard, writes frequently about health-care issues. This book on improving patient safety explains some of the basic approaches to a critical issue. He also writes frequently for the *New Yorker*. In the following article, he details how other developed countries created their health-care systems to ensure universal coverage beginning after World War II: "Getting There from Here: How Should Obama Reform Health Care?," *New Yorker*, January 26, 2009, 26–33.

Linda Kohn, Janet Corrigan, and Molla Donaldson, eds. *To Err Is Human: Building a Safer Health System.* Washington, DC: National Academy Press, 1999.

> This now classic book from the staff of the Institute of Medicine opened the eyes of the medical world to the issue of patient safety in medicine, noting that about 100,000 die each year from preventable medical errors and presenting some logical and sensible approaches for improving safety.

T. R. Reid. *The Healing of America: A Global Quest for Better, Cheaper, and Fairer Health Care.* New York: Penguin Press, 2009.

> Reid is a correspondent for the *Washington Post* and National Public Radio. Aware that America is the only country in the developed world where access to health care is not universal, he traveled to multiple countries and used an old shoulder injury as rationale to visit doctors in each locale to learn firsthand how medicine is practiced differently than it is in the United States. In the process he developed his view on how America should reform its system of care by borrowing ideas from other countries.

Stephen C. Schimpff. *The Future of Medicine: Megatrends in Health Care That Will Improve Your Quality of Life.* Nashville, TN: Thomas Nelson, 2007.

> This companion volume to the present book explains the remarkable changes coming in medical care as a result of scientific advances in fields such as genomics, stem cells, vaccines, medical devices, imaging, the operating room, and many others.

Staff of the *Washington Post*. *Landmark: The Inside Story of America's New Health Care Law and What It Means for Us All.* New York: Public Affairs, 2010.

The *Washington Post* reporters who covered the health-care debate in Congress wrote a useful book on what the final legislation means for doctors, hospitals, insurers, and the American public. It also offers fresh insights into the battles among members of Congress, the president's staff, and the multiple lobbying groups, all of whom had an important impact on the final legislation.

H. Gilbert Welch, Lisa M. Schwartz, and Steven Woloshin. *Overdiagnosed: Making People Sick in the Pursuit of Health.* Boston: Beacon Press, 2011.

Somewhat along the same theme as Shannon Brownlee's book, Welsh, Schwartz, and Woloshin suggest that there is far too much testing of asymptomatic individuals. It raises total health-care expenditures, leads to way too many interventions and procedures that are not necessary, and occasionally causes real harm. This message is consistent with many of the patients' stories I describe in this volume.

Professional Journals

Many professional journals publish useful articles on health-care delivery; however, these three devote substantial space to high-quality, peer-reviewed articles on a regular basis.

Health Affairs (http://www.healthaffairs.org) is the leading monthly journal on health policy issues. It tends to develop a specific topic in depth in each issue. The June 2011 issue, for example, is devoted to the global opportunities for massively reducing morbidity and mortality at relatively low cost with vaccines.

Journal of the American Medical Association (http://jama.ama-assn.org), one of the most widely read medical journals, regularly publishes articles on health-care delivery and health-care reform.

New England Journal of Medicine (http://www.nejm.org), arguably the most respected of all medical journals, has published one or more articles on health-care reform or other related policy issues nearly every week for the past few years. Perusal of the online archives reveals a wealth of useful and interesting articles under the heading "Perspectives."

Government Agencies

Centers for Disease Control and Prevention (http://www.cdc.gov) has as its mission "to collaborate to create the expertise, information, and tools that people and communities need to protect their health—through health promotion, prevention of disease, injury and disability, and preparedness for new health threats." Its website is a wealth of useful information about vaccines, health promotion, and disease prevention and has many excellent interactive graphics on subjects such as the increasing threat of obesity and the quickly increasing epidemic of diabetes.

CDC leaders Ali H. Mokdad, J. S. Marks, D. F. Stroup, and J. L. Gerberding published the eye-opening piece "Actual Causes of Death in the United States, 2000," *Journal of American Medical Association* 291, no. 10 (2004): 1238–45. We usually think of death as caused by an illness such as heart disease, cancer, or stroke, but they are often the end result of other factors that preceded them, such as obesity and smoking. This article spells out what these predisposing factors are, demonstrating that in large part most are owing to our lifestyle and behaviors.

National Institutes of Health (http://www.nih.gov) is the nation's (and world's) pre-eminent medical research agency. Headquartered in Bethesda, Maryland, it has an annual budget of more than $31 billion. It distributes about 80 percent of its funding through grants to more than 325,000 scientists at universities, medical schools, and research institutions across the country based on peer-reviewed scientific proposals. Its 6,000 in-house scientists also engage in critical research on pressing issues, and its Bethesda hospital, The Clinical Center (http://clinical-center.nih.gov), serves as the world's largest hospital devoted entirely to medical research. The NIH comprises multiple institutes, each focused on one or more specific area of research, such as:

> The National Cancer Institute (http://www.cancer.gov)
> The National Heart Lung and Blood Institute (http://www.nhlbi.nih.gov)
> The National Institute of Allergy and Infectious Diseases (http://www.niaid.nih.gov)

Their websites are filled with useful information that has the advantage of being carefully reviewed to be sure it is scientifically based and valid. You can access any of them from the main NIH website.

State, county, and city health departments maintain websites where you can obtain relevant and up-to-date information about local programs.

Hospitals

Most hospitals' websites are primarily devoted to information on their own programs, physicians who practice there, and directions for visits. A few of the larger hospitals, usually academic medical centers, have extensive health-related websites that include substantial information about new medical discoveries and treatment approaches. In general, they do not address health-care delivery issues.

A word of caution: The old-time "snake oil" salesmen have not disappeared. If you are searching for information about a particular disease, remember that the Web is full of sites touting unproven methodologies or seeking your money for useless information. You should confine your search to the sites of reputable organizations, such as those listed here, other major well-known academic medical centers, and the National Institutes of Health or the Centers for Disease Control and Prevention.

The Mayo Clinic (http://www.mayoclinic.com) and the Cleveland Clinic (http://my .clevelandclinic.org) have excellent sites for garnering knowledge about specific disease conditions and health promotion approaches. All of their information listed is well founded.

University of Maryland Medical Center's website (http://www.umm.edu) has become one of the most visited hospital sites. It is an excellent source of information on myriad diseases and medical issues. The content is based on the School of Medicine's faculty input.

Nonprofit Organizations, Foundations, Associations, and Washington Think Tanks

Many nonprofit agencies specialize in health-related issues. As health care has become a major topic for Congress, many Washington-based organizations seek either to influence congressional or government agency decision making or to inform the public of the complexities of health-care delivery. Here are a few.

The American Hospital Association (http://www.aha.org) represents the nation's over 5000 hospitals with a vision for healthy communities. It is an active advocacy organization for the interests of its constituents.

The Association of American Medical Colleges (https://www.aamc.org) represents the medical schools and their affiliated teaching hospitals.

The Henry J. Kaiser Family Foundation (http://www.kff.org) serves "as a non-partisan source of facts, information, and analysis for policymakers, the media, the health care community, and the public. Our product is information, always provided free of charge." The foundation's polls on Americans' sentiments toward the health reform legislation are excellent; I referred to them frequently in chapter 7. The foundation also maintains a major Web-based health news and information service.

The Heritage Foundation is a conservative foundation with a substantial commitment to health-care delivery policy (http://www.heritage.org/initiatives/health-care). It seeks to transform insurance products so that they are more fully controlled by the individual purchasers. Individuals will take a more active role in their health-care expenditures by having a greater control of the dollars expended on their behalf.

The Institute of Medicine (http://www.iom.edu) of the National Academies is chartered by Congress to provide unbiased advice to decision makers in government and the private sector about health and health care.

The New America Foundation (http://health.newamerica.net) is a nonprofit, nonpartisan foundation that "emphasizes work that is responsive to the changing conditions and problems of our 21st Century information-age economy—an era shaped by transforming innovation and wealth creation, but also by shortened job tenures, longer life spans, mobile capital, financial imbalances and rising inequality." It has long had a major interest in health-care delivery issues. It focused previously on increasing access and is now geared more toward increasing quality and cost effectiveness.

The Robert Wood Johnson Foundation (http://www.rwjf.org) is devoted to health policy and improved health-care delivery. It makes grants to individuals and organizations to address certain areas at their root causes such as childhood obesity and public health.

Organizations Focused on Specific Diseases or Treatments

A vast number of nonprofit organizations focus on a single disease or group of diseases. The larger ones have extensive consumer information, all available on their websites. Here are just a few. Again, remember that there are many disreputable sites suggesting unproven remedies. Avoid them.

The American Cancer Society (http://www.cancer.org) is dedicated to both the prevention and treatment of cancer. It also lobbies for insurance coverage of effective screening, treatment, and early diagnostic modalities. The latter activities brought the ACS into the health reform debate.

The American Heart Association (http://www.heart.org), which is combined with the American Stroke Association, is dedicated to reducing the impact of cardiovascular disease on the world's population. As such the groups provide excellent information on nutrition, weight management, stress reduction, and smoking cessation along with more detailed information on preventing cardiovascular disease. They also offer classes on cardiopulmonary resuscitation (CPR) along with other health classes.

The Juvenile Diabetes Foundation (http://www.jdrf.org) was founded in 1970 by parents of children with type 1 diabetes primarily to fund research for finding a cure. It remains the foundation's principal activity.

INDEX

Academic Medical Centers (AMCs), 28,
   82–83, 184–86, 187, 188
access to medical care
   Americans and, 3–4, 15, 17, 66, 199
   costs, 26
   insurance restrictions, 52
   patient expectations, 53–54
   personal responsibility and, 195–97
   reform vision and proposal, 19, 31,
      37, 216, 224–25
accountability
   in care systems, 8, 106, 125, 171–72
   for errors, 131, 132, 218–19
accountable care organizations (ACOs),
   171–72, 181, 205
acid reflux, 117–18
acid suppressors, 87–88, 117–18, 120,
   135–36
"Actual Cause of Death in the United
   States, 2000" (Mokdad), 13–14, 242
acupuncture, 46–47, 69, 146, 173
adjunct providers, use of, 34, 64, 169–70,
   171, 177, 222
administrative fees, 65, 165
administrative waste, 23–24, 145, 153,
   212, 224
advertising, 113–14, 116–17, 119, 136, 187
Aetna, 147, 180, 200
Affordable Health Care Act
   accountable care organizations,
      171–72
   bundled payment program, 159–60
   catastrophic illness, 149

comparative effectiveness research,
   217, 237n4
concerns and deficiencies, 85, 94–95,
   193, 197, 202–3
elements of, 17, 95, 154, 202–7, 241
Medicare, 95, 104, 173
passing of, 198–99, 241
philosophy of, 197
public opinion, 203
aging population, 18, 22, 50, 96, 114–15,
   169, 222
agriculture, 37, 111, 187
AIDS, 35, 43
air systems in hospitals, 129
Aisner, Joseph, 235n4
alcohol use, 13–14, 117, 135
*All I Really Need to Know I Learned in
   Kindergarten* (Fulghum), 185
Alzheimer's disease, 37, 43, 112
AMCs. *See* Academic Medical Centers
American Cancer Society (ACS), 146, 244
American Heart Association, 244
American Hospital Association, 243
American Recovery and Reinvestment
   Acts, 121, 200, 237n4
amoxicillin, 87
angioplasty, 72, 121–22, 143
animals and organ transplants, 44
Anne Arundel Medical Center, 70
antibiotics
   historical use, 4, 5
   home-based therapy, 173
   hospital-acquired infections, 24

ABOUT THE AUTHOR

Stephen C. Schimpff, MD, received his BA degree from Rutgers University and his medical degree from Yale, where he remained for his internal medicine residency training. He joined the Baltimore Cancer Research Center at the National Cancer Institute (NCI), where he was trained in both medical oncology and infectious diseases. He is board certified in internal medicine, medical oncology, and infectious diseases. For thirteen years at NCI, he cared for patients with leukemia and lymphomas and conducted research into the serious infectious diseases that beset cancer patients. In 1982 he was appointed founding director of what is now the University of Maryland Marlene and Stewart Greenebaum Cancer Center and in 1985 was recruited to become executive vice president and chief operating officer of the University of Maryland Medical System, now a twelve-hospital system. In 1999 he became chief executive officer of the University of Maryland Medical Center, the system's flagship academic tertiary care hospital. Schimpff is a professor at the University of Maryland's School of Medicine and School of Public Policy.

Schimpff has been active in numerous civic groups and professional associations and served as chair of the board of governors of the National Institutes of Health Clinical Center. He has published more than two hundred scientific articles, reviews, book chapters, and editorials, and edited three medical texts. Since quasi-retirement in 2004 he has authored *The Future of Medicine: Megatrends in Health Care That Will Improve Your Quality of Life* and coauthored *Alignment: The Key to Success of the University of Maryland Medical System.* His website is www.medicalmega trends.com and his blog is at http://medicalmegatrends.blogspot.com.

He and Carol, his wife of forty-eight years, live in Columbia, Maryland, and enjoy visiting their cabin in Canaan Valley, West Virginia, where they volunteer at the Canaan Valley National Wildlife Refuge. They also travel to Studio City, California, where their daughter, son-in-law, and two wonderful grandchildren reside.